2

Biochemistry of

Antimicrobial Action

Biochemistry of Antimicrobial Action

Third Edition

T.J. FRANKLIN and G.A. SNOW

Imperial Chemical Industries Ltd,
Pharmaceuticals Division, Alderley Park,
Macclesfield, Cheshire

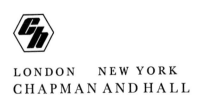

LONDON   NEW YORK
CHAPMAN AND HALL

First published 1971
by Chapman and Hall Ltd.,
11 New Fetter Lane, London EC4P 4EE
Second edition 1975
Third edition 1981
Published in the USA by
Chapman and Hall
in association with Methuen, Inc.
733 Third Avenue, New York, NY 10017

© *1981 T.J. Franklin and G.A. Snow*

Printed in Great Britain at the
University Printing House, Cambridge

ISBN 0 412 22440 2 (cased)
ISBN 0 412 22450 X (paperback)

British Library Cataloguing in Publication Data

Franklin, Trevor John
    Biochemistry of antimicrobial action. — 3rd ed.
    1. Anti-infective agents
    I. Title   II. Snow, Geroge Alan
    615'.7   RM263   80-41090

    ISBN 0-412-22440-2
    ISBN 0-412-22450-X Pbk

Contents

Preface   *page x*
Preface to the third edition   *xii*

1 **The development of antimicrobial agents, past, present and future**   1
   The social and economic importance of antimicrobial agents   1
   An outline of the historical development of antimicrobial agents and of
   chemotherapeutic theories   2
     Early remedies   2
     Antiseptics and disinfectants   3
     The beginnings of chemotherapy   4
     The debt of chemotherapy to Ehrlich   6
     The treatment of bacterial infections by synthetic compounds   9
     The antibiotic revolution   10
   Reasons for studying the biochemistry of antimicrobial compounds   12
   Development of biochemical knowledge of antimicrobial action   13
     Pharmacological biochemistry   13
     Nature of the biochemical systems affected   14
     *Methods used for the study of the mode of action of antimicrobial
   compounds*   14
     Selectivity of action of antimicrobial agents   17
     *The molecular interaction between the antimicrobial agent and the
   target site*   17
     The biochemistry of microbial resistance   18
   Scope and layout of the present book   19

2 **The bacterial cell wall - a vulnerable shield**   21
   Functions of the wall   21
   Wall structure   21
     The Gram-positive wall   22
     The Gram-negative wall   24
   Structure and biosynthesis of peptidoglycan   28
     Stage 1. *Synthesis of UDP-N-acetylmuramic acid*   29
     Stage 2. *Building the pentapeptide side chain*   29
     Stage 3. *Membrane-bound reactions leading to a linear*   30
     peptidoglycan polymer
     Stage 4. *Cross-linking*   33
     Variations in peptidoglycan structure   35

page

Cross-linking in Gram-negative bacteria 35
Attachments to peptidoglycans 36
Antibiotics having a primary action on peptidoglycan biosynthesis ... 38
Phosphomycin (Phosphonomycin) 39
Cycloserine 39
Vancomycin, enduracidin, moenomycin and tunicamycin 41
Penicillins, cephalosporins and other β-lactam antibotics 43
Site of action of penicillins and cephalosporins 47
Actions of β-lactam antibacterials on Gram-negative bacteria ... 52
Bacitracin 53
Other antibiotics affecting wall synthesis 55
Cerulenin 55
Polyoxins - inhibitors of fungal wall synthesis 56

3 Antiseptics, antibiotics and the cell membrane 58
Bacteria killers: antiseptics and disinfectants 58
Phenols 60
Cationic antiseptics 61
Polypeptide antibiotics 64
Ionophoric antibiotics 67
Pore-forming antibiotics 73
Gramicidin A 73
The polyene antibiotics 75

**4 Suppression of gene function 1. Inhibitors of the synthesis of
nucleic acids** 79
Types of inhibitor of nucleic acid synthesis 80
Inhibitors of the biosynthesis of nucleotide precursors 80
Azaserine and 6-diazo-5-oxo-L-norleucine (DON) 80
Hadacidin 82
Psicofuranine and decoyinine 83
Mycophenolic acid 84
Inhibitors of nucleic acid synthesis at the polymerization level 85
A. Intercalating compounds 86
Acridines, phenanthridines and chloroquine 88
Actinomycin D 89
Intercalation of actinomycin D 90
Bifunctional intercalating drugs: the quinoxaline antibiotics . 92
Bleomycins: DNA-strand-breaking drugs that may intercalate . 94
Inhibition of nucleic acid synthesis by drugs that intercalate . 95
B. Cross-linkers of DNA: mitomycin and porfiromycin 95
C. Drugs that inhibit nucleic acid polymerases 97
Inhibitors of RNA polymerase: rifamycins, streptovaricins
and streptolydigin 97
Inhibitors of DNA polymerase 102
Hydroxyphenylazopyrimidines 102
Nalidixic acid 104
Novobiocin 105
Inhibition of nucleic acid synthesis by drugs that become
incorporated into the DNA template 106

page

5-Iododeoxyuridine (IdUrd)   106
Arabinosyl cytosine and arabinosyl adenine   107

5   **Suppression of gene function 2. Interference with the translation of the genetic message: inhibitors of protein synthesis**   110
Ribosomes   110
Stages in protein biosynthesis   111
   Formation of aminoacyl-transfer RNA   111
   Initiation   113
   Peptide bond synthesis and chain elongation   114
   Chain termination and release   115
Puromycin   115
Inhibitors of aminoacyl transfer RNA formation   117
Inhibitors of initiation-complex formation and transfer
RNA-ribsome interaction   118
   Streptomycin   118
      Specificity and site of action of streptomycin   118
   Other aminoglycoside antibiotics   121
   Tetracylines   123
Inhibitors of peptide bond formation and translocation   126
   Chloramphenicol   126
   Erythromycin   128
   Lincomycin and clindamycin   130
   Fusidic acid   131
   Cycloheximide   132
Some effects of inhibitors of protein synthesis on living cells   132
   Prokaryotic cells   132
      Effect of inhibitors of protein synthesis on polysomes   133
      Nucleic acid synthesis during inhibition of protein synthesis   134
Effects of inhibitors of 70S ribosomes on eukaryotic cells   135

6   **Synthetic antimicrobial agents and compounds with special applications**   138
The sulphonamide antibacterials   138
Antagonists of dihydrofolate reductase   142
Antimicrobial agents affecting terminal respiration   145
   Antimycin   145
   Carboxin and piericidin   147
   Oligomycin   147
Other antibacterial agents   149
   Quinoxaline and phenazine N-oxides   149
   The nitrofuran antibacterials   150
   Isonicotinic hydrazide (INH)   150
   Sideromycins   150
Antifungal agents   151
   Fungicides affecting sterol biosynthesis   152
   Griseofulvin and benomyl   152
Compounds used in treating protozoal diseases   154
Chemotherapy of virus diseases   156

page

7 **Penetrating the defences: how antimicrobial agents reach their targets**   159
Cellular permeability barriers to drug penetration   159
   The cytoplasmic membrane   159
      Passive diffusion   160
      Facilitated diffusion   161
   The outer layers of bacterial cells   162
      Pore structure of the outer membrane of Gram-negative bacteria   164
Some examples of modes of penetration of antibacterial drugs   165
   Passive diffusion   165
   Facilitated diffusion   166
      D-Cycloserine   166
      Tetracyclines   166
      Sideromycins   167
      Streptomycin   168
      Phosophomycin   168
The exploitation of transport systems in the design of new antimicrobial agents   169

8 **The problems of resistance to antimicrobial drugs**   172
The genetics of drug resistance   172
The nature of genetic alterations that give rise to drug-resistant variants   173
   Spontaneous mutations   173
Spread of drug-resistance by the transfer of genetic information   174
   Transformation   174
   Transduction   174
   Conjugation and R-factors   177
      Transposons   178
      Molecular properties of R-factors   179
      The conjugation process   181
      Clinical importance of R-factors   183
Biochemical mechanisms of drug-resistance   184
   Summary of possible mechanisms   184
   (1) Conversion of an active drug to an in-active derivative   185
      Inactivation of β-lactam antibiotics   185
      Gram-negative β-lactamases   186
      Chemical approaches to the β-lactamase problem   187
      Origin of β-lactamases   188
      Inactivation of chloroamphenicol by acetylation   189
      Physiology of chloramphenicol acetyltransferase synthesis   190
      Comparison of chloramphenicol acetyltransferases from Gram-positive and Gram-negative cells   191
      Inactivation of aminoglycoside antibiotics   192
   (2) Modification of the drug-sensitive site   194
      Streptomycin   194
      Kasugamycin   195
      Erythromycin   195
      Rifamycins   195
   (3) Loss of cell permeability to a drug   196

page

(4) Provision of an alternative enzyme or pathway that bypasses the
  inhibited reaction — 198
(5) Increased production of a drug-sensitive enzyme. — 200
(6) Increased production of a metabolite that antagonizes the
  inhibitor — 201
(7) Decreased requirement for the product of an inhibited
  reaction — 201
Practical approaches to the control of drug-resistance — 201

Index — 205

Cover Photograph

The micrograph is taken from *J. Infect. Dis.*, **128** (1973) 793
and is reproduced here with the kind permission of the authors,
D. Greenwood and F. O'Grady, and The University of Chicago
Press. It shows the effect of 10 μg/ml of Mecillinam on
E. coli visualized by scanning electron microscopy after 60
min treatment. See also Fig. 2.18.

Preface

The rapid advances made in the study of the synthesis, structure and function of biological macromolecules in the last fifteen years have enabled scientists concerned with antimicrobial agents to achieve a considerable measure of understanding of how these substances inhibit cell growth and division. The use of antimicrobial agents as highly specific inhibitors has in turn substantially assisted the investigation of complex biochemical processes. The literature in this field is so extensive however, that we considered an attempt should be made to draw together in an introductory book the more significant studies of recent years. This book, which is in fact based on lecture courses given by us to undergraduates at Liverpool and Manchester Universities, is therefore intended as an introduction to the biochemistry of antimicrobial action for advanced students in many disciplines. We hope that it may also be useful to established scientists who are new to this area of research.

The book is concerned with a discussion of medically important antimicrobial compounds and also a number of agents that, although having no medical uses, have proved invaluable as research tools in biochemistry. Our aim has been to present the available information in a simple and readable way, emphasizing the established facts rather than more controversial material. Whenever possible, however, we have indicated the gaps in the present knowledge of the subject where further information is required. We have avoided the use of literature references in the text; instead we have included short lists of key articles and books for further reading at the end of each chapter.

We have drawn on the work of many scientists and we are especially pleased to express our thanks to those who have given us permission to reproduce their original diagrams and photographs. We are also grateful to the Pharmaceuticals Division of Imperial Chemicals Industries Ltd, for providing the necessary facilities for the preparation of this book.

Abbreviations used without definition for common biochemical substances are those recommended by the Biochemical Journal (1970).

June 1970

T.J. FRANKLIN
G. A. SNOW

Preface to the third edition

During the period since the appearance of the second edition there have been some important advances in the biochemistry of anti-bacterial action which this new edition attempts to cover. Most notable, perhaps, has been the explosion of interest in β-lactam drugs. Many new semisynthetic and naturally occurring members of this group have appeared and there has been renewed vigour in research into both the mode of action of, and resistance to, β-lactams. In other directions advances have been significant though less spectacular. Further research has resolved some areas of doubt and has placed the mode of action of many compounds on a sounder basis. The new information has necessitated extensive rewriting of every chapter except the first, and reference is made to some twenty-seven more antimicrobial compounds than in the last edition. To ensure the continuity of the text we have again chosen to confine the literature references to the ends of chapters. The reading lists have been extended, updated and subdivided according to major headings.

T. J. FRANKLIN
G. A. SNOW

May 1980

1 The development of antimicrobial agents, past, present and future

The social and economic importance of antimicrobial agents

Few developments in the history of medicine have had such a profound effect upon human life and society as the development of the power to control infections due to micro-organisms. The impact has been felt in many ways. We in the advanced countries have been freed from the devastating plagues that in earlier days decimated the population leaving a trail of misery and social disruption. No longer is surgery a desperate gamble with human life. The perils of childbirth are greatly lessened with the control of puerperal fever. The death of children and young adults from meningitis, tuberculosis and septicaemia, once a commonplace is now a rarity. All these benefits are now accepted without question, but they have changed the fabric of our lives. The control of infectious disease has also brought is own social and medical problems. Within our own highly developed society the conquest of pneumonia, sometimes called 'the old man's friend', has helped to raise the expectation of life. People live longer and the aged form an increasing part of our population.

The ability to control infectious disease has emphasized our lesser success in dealing with degenerative diseases, and an extended life span is a dubious advantage if it is accompanied by failing faculties and the feeling of being a burden on an uncaring society. In the poorer and less-developed countries the control of infection has begun to show its effects. Nearly all the diseases affecting many millions of people, such as tuberculosis, malaria, leprosy and schistosomiasis could in principle be abolished or reduced to minor proportions. The only substantial obstacle to achieving this is the cost. The continued prevalence of these diseases is a reflection on the disparity still remaining between the 'haves' and the 'have nots'. Even so, considerable progress has been made. The most obvious result is a sudden increase in populations. Communities where endemic disease and periodic plagues previously kept the death rate in balance with the birth rate are now expanding at an alarming rate. This effect may well increase as measures against infection improve. Population control may be essential if these communities are not to suffer the effects of gross overcrowding and undernourishment in place of their previous situation of high maternal and infantile mortality and short life expectation due to infectious disease.

In the fight against infectious disease several factors have combined to produce the remarkable achievements already outlined. The first advances were mainly the result of improved sanitation and housing. These removed some of the worst foci of infectious disease and limited the spread of infection through vermin and insect parasites or by contaminated water and food. The earliest effective direct control of infectious diseases was achieved through vaccination and similar immunological methods. These still play a large part in the control of infection today, and they are the mainstay of our attack on virus diseases which largely resist treatment by chemotherapeutic agents. The use of antimicrobial drugs for control of infection is almost entirely a development of this century, and the most dramatic developments have taken place only since the late 1930s. The practical importance of antimicrobial agents is enormous. In the pharmaceutical industry this is probably the largest class of drugs with world sales around £4000m per annum (1979). Rarely has so complete a success been achieved in the medical field in so short a time. Before describing the biochemistry underlying the action of antimicrobial drugs we shall consider the work that made these drugs available to us and the thought that lay behind their discovery.

An outline of the historical development of antimicrobial agents and of chemotherapeutic theories

Early remedies

Among the many traditional and folk remedies two sources of antimicrobial compounds have survived to the present day. These are cinchona bark for the treatment of malaria and ipecacuanha root for amoebic dysentery. Cinchona bark was used by the Indians of Peru for treating malaria and was introduced into European medicine by the Spaniards in the early seventeenth century. The active principle, quinine, was isolated in 1820. Quinine remained the only treatment for malaria until well into the twentieth century and still has a place in chemotherapy. Ipecacuanha root was known in Brazil and probably in Asia for its curative action in diarrhoeas and dysentery. Emetine was isolated as the active constituent in 1817 and was shown in 1891 to have a specific action against amoebic dysentery. It is still used for treating this disease. These early remedies were used along with many ineffectual nostrums without any understanding of the nature of the diseases. Malaria, for example, was thought to be caused by miasmas arising from marshy places; the significance of the blood-borne parasite was not recognized until 1883 and only in 1899 was the anophelene mosquito proved to be the specific insect vector.

Antiseptics and disinfectants

The use of disinfectants and antiseptics also preceded understanding of their action, and seems to have arisen from the observation that certain substances stopped putrefaction of meat or rotting of wood. The term 'antiseptic' itself was apparently first used by Pringle in 1750 to describe substances that prevent putrefaction. The idea was eventually applied to the treatment of suppurating wounds. Mercuric chloride was used by Arabian physicians in the Middle Ages for preventing sepsis in open wounds. However, it was not until the nineteenth century that antiseptics came into general use in medicine. Chlorinated soda, essentially hypochlorite, was introduced in 1825 by Labarraque for the treatment of infected wounds, and tincture of iodine was first used in 1839. One of the earliest examples of disinfection used in preventing the spread of infectious disease was recorded by Oliver Wendel Holmes in 1835. He regularly washed his hands in a solution of chloride of lime when dealing with cases of puerperal fever and thereby greatly reduced the incidence of fresh infections. These pioneer attempts at antisepsis were not generally accepted until Pasteur's publication in 1863 of the microbial origin of putrefaction. This led to an understanding of the origin of infection and suggested the rationale of its prevention. As so often in the history of medicine a change of practice depended upon the personality and persistence of one man. In antiseptics this man was Lister. He took phenol, the antiseptic which had been introduced by Lemaire in 1860, and applied it vigorously in surgery. A 2.5 per cent solution was used for dressing wounds and twice this concentration for sterilizing instruments. Later he used a spray of phenol solution to produce an essentially sterile environment for carrying out surgical operations. The previous state of surgery had been deplorable; wounds usually became infected and the mortality rate was appalling. The effect of Lister's measures was revolutionary, and the antiseptic technique opened the way to great surgical advances. Even at this time, about 1870, the use of antiseptics was still empirical. An understanding of their function began with the work of Koch who from 1881 onwards introduced the techniques on which modern bacteriology has been built. He perfected methods of obtaining pure cultures of bacteria and of growing them on solid media, and he demonstrated practical methods of sterile working. Once it became possible to handle bacteria in a controlled environment the action of disinfectants and antiseptics could be studied. The pioneer work on the scientific approach to this subject was published by Kronig and Paul in 1897.

Since that time the history of antiseptics has been of steady but unspectacular improvement. Many of the traditional antiseptics have continued in use in refined forms. The phenols have been modified and made more acceptable for general use. Acriflavine, introduced in 1913, was the first of a number of basic antiseptics. It had many years of use but has been largely displaced in the last three decades by colourless cationic antiseptics. In surgery the antiseptic era gave place to the aseptic era in which the emphasis was on the avoidance of bacterial contamination rather than on killing bacteria already present. All the same, infection of surgical wounds is a constant risk and antiseptics are still used as an extra precaution or second line of defence. Disinfectants also play an important part in the hygiene of milking sheds, broiler houses and other places where strict asepsis is impracticable.

The beginnings of chemotherapy

The publications of Pasteur and Koch firmly established that micro-organisms are the cause of infectious disease, though for some diseases the causative organism still remained to be discovered. It was also known that bacteria are killed by various antiseptics and disinfectants. Not surprisingly attempts were made to kill micro-organisms within the body and so to end an infection. Koch himself carried out some experiments with this aim. He had shown the action of mercuric chloride against the anthrax bacillus; it is one of the few disinfectants that kill the particularly tough spores of this organism. He therefore tried to cure animals of anthrax infection by injecting mercuric chloride. Unfortunately the animals died of mercury poisoning and their organs still contained infectious anthrax bacilli. A slightly more successful attempt to cure an infection with a toxic agent was made by Lindgard in 1893. He treated horses suffering from *surra*, a disease now known to be caused by trypanosome, with arsenious oxide. There was some improvement of the disease, but the compound was too toxic to be generally useful.

Chemotherapy however really began with Paul Ehrlich. During the ten years from 1902 onwards Ehrlich's work foreshadowed almost all the concepts which have governed subsequent work on synthetic antimicrobial agents. His first ideas arose from studies with 'vital stains': dyestuffs that were taken up selectively by living tissue. One such dye was methylene blue, which in the animal body is concentrated in nervous tissue. Ehrlich showed that the same dye was readily taken up by the malaria parasites in the blood, so that they become deeply stained. Consequently methylene blue was tried against human malaria and showed some effect, though not sufficient to make it a useful treatment. Nevertheless this minor success started a line of thought that was to prove of the greatest significance. Ehrlich believed that antimicrobial agents must be essentially toxic compounds and that they must bind to the micro-organism in order to exert their action. The problem was to discover compounds having a selective action against the microbial cell compared with the cells of the host animal. Starting from methylene blue Ehrlich began to search for other dyestuffs that would affect protozoal diseases. In 1904, after testing hundreds of available dyes, he eventually found one that was effective against trypanosomiasis in horses. This compound called trypan red was a significant landmark in the treatment of microbial infections since it was the first man-made compound that produced a curative effect.

However, it was not in the field of dyestuffs that Ehrlich achieved his greatest success. Following the early work on the treatment of trypanosomiasis with arsenious oxide, Koch tested the organic arsenical atoxyl (Fig. 1.1). This compound produced the first cures of sleeping sickness, a human trypanosomal disease. The compound however produced unfortunate side effects, some patients developing optic atrophy. The curative successs of this compound stimulated Ehrlich to make other related arsenicals. He tested these on mice infected experimentally with trypanosomiasis, and showed that curative action did not run parallel with toxicity to the mice. This suggested that if enough compounds were made some would have sufficiently low toxicity to be safe as chemotherapeutic agents. Ehrlich continued his search for compounds active against various micro-organisms and showed that arsenicals were active against the causative organism of syphilis. He began a massive search for an organoarsenical compound that could be used in the treatment of this disease and eventually in 1910 discovered the famous drug salvarsan (Fig. 1.1). This drug and its derivative neo-salvarsan became the standard treatment for syphilis. Coupled with bismuth therapy they remained in use until supplanted by penicillin in 1945. This was the most spectacular practical achievement of Ehrlich's career, but

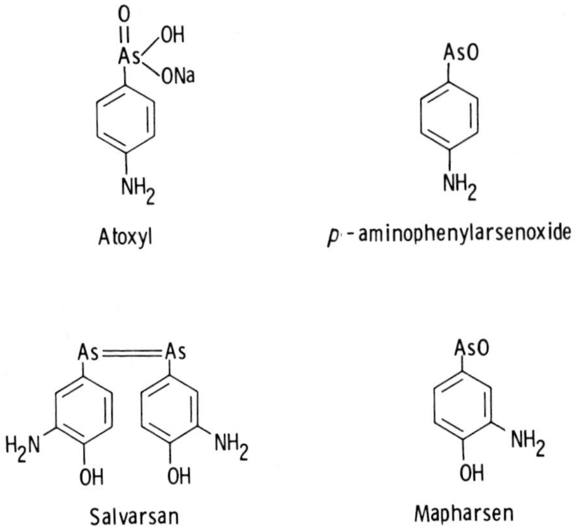

Figure 1.1 Arsenical compounds used in the treatment of trypanosomiasis or syphilis.

scientifically he is remembered at least as much for his wealth of ideas that have inspired workers in the field of chemotherapy down to the present day. These ideas are so important that they deserve separate consideration.

The debt of chemotherapy to Ehrlich

The very term *chemotherapy* was invented by Ehrlich and expressed his belief that infectious disease could be combated by treatment with synthetic chemicals. Successes since his day have entirely justified his faith in this possibility. He postulated that cells possess chemical receptors which are concerned with the uptake of nutrients. Drugs that affect the cell must bind to one or other of these receptors. The toxicity of a drug is determined firstly by its distribution in the body. However, in the treatment of an infection it is the binding to the parasite relative to the host cell that determines the effectiveness of the compound. Thus Ehrlich recognized the importance of quantitative measurement of the relationship between the dose of a compound required to produce a therapeutic effect and the dose that will cause toxic reactions. Such measurements are still of prime importance in chemotherapy today. Ehrlich's view of cell receptors also has its counterpart in modern views of membrane transport.

Ehrlich pioneered methods that have since become the mainstay of the search for new drugs. One aspect of his approach was the use of 'screening'. This is the application of a relatively simple test to large numbers of compounds in order to obtain evidence of biological activity in types of chemical structure not previously examined. The second of Ehrlich's methods was the deliberate synthesis of chemical variants of a compound known to have the required activity. The new compounds were examined for increased activity or for improvements in some other property such as reduced toxicity. Any improvement found was used as a guide to further synthesis eventually arriving, by a series of steps, at the best possible compound. These methods are now so well-accepted that their novelty in Ehrlich's day can easily be forgotten. They depend on the thesis that a useful drug possesses an ideal combination of structural features which cannot be predicted at the outset. A compound having a sufficiently close structural approximation will show some degree of activity, and can therefore act as a 'lead' towards the best attainable structure.

According to Ehrlich a chemotherapeutic substance has two functional features, the 'haptophore' or binding group which enables the compound to attach itself to the cell receptors, and the 'toxophore' or toxic group that brings about an adverse effect on the cell. This idea has had a continuing influence in subsequent years. In cancer chemotherapy it has frequently been used in attempts to bring about specific concentration of toxic agents or antimetabolites in tumour cells. In antimicrobial research it has helped to explain some features of the biochemical action of antimicrobial compounds. The action of the sideromycins may well be interpreted in terms of a haptophoric and toxophoric group (Chapter 6).

Ehrlich also recognized that compounds acting on microbial infection need not necessarily kill the invading organism. It was, he suggested, sufficient to prevent substantial multiplication of the infectious agent, since the normal body defences, antibodies and phagocytes would cope with foreign organisms provided that their numbers were not overwhelming. His views on this topic were based in part on his observation that isolated spirochetes treated with low concentrations of salvarsan remained motile and were therefore apparently still alive. Nevertheless they were unable to produce an infection when they were injected into an animal body. It is a striking fact that many of today's important antibacterial drugs are bacteriostatic rather than bactericidal.

Another feature of Ehrlich's work was his recognition of the possibility that drugs may be activated by metabolism in the body. This suggestion was prompted by the observation that the compound atoxyl was active against trypanosomal infections but was inactive against isolated trypanosomes. His explanation was that atoxyl was reduced in the body to the much more toxic *p*-aminophenyl-arsenoxide (Fig. 1.1). More recent work shows that atoxyl and other related arsonic acids are not readily reduced to arsenoxides in the body; however, local reduction by the parasite remains a possibility. Ehrlich, surprisingly, did not recognize that his own compound salvarsan would undergo metabolic cleavage. In animals it gives rise to the arsenoxide as the first of a series of metabolites. This compound was introduced into medicine in 1932 under the name mapharsen (Fig. 1.1); its toxicity is rather high, but it has sufficient selectivity to give it useful chemotherapeutic properties. Several other examples of activation through metabolism have been dis-covered in more recent times. The most notable perhaps are the reduction of Prontosil rubrum to sulphanilamide and the conversion of proguanil to the active dihydrotriazine (Chapter 6).

Ehrlich also drew attention to the problem of resistance of micro-organisms towards chemotherapeutic compounds. He noticed it in the treatment of trypanosomes with parafuchsin and later with trypan red and atoxyl. He found that resistance extended to other compounds chemically related to the original three, but there was no cross-resistance between the groups. In Ehrlich's view this was evidence that each of these compounds was affecting a separate receptor. Independent resistance to different drugs later became a commonplace in antimicrobial therapy. Ehrlich's view of the nature of resistance is also interesting. He found that trypanosomes resistant to trypan red absorbed less of the dyestuff than sensitive strains, and he postulated that the receptors in resistant organisms had a diminished affinity for the dye. This mechanism corresponds to one of the currently accepted types of resistance in micro-organisms (Chapter 8).

Several useful antimicrobial drugs arose in later years as an extension of Ehrlich's work. The most notable are suramin, a develop-ment from trypan red, and mepacrine (also known as quinacrine or atebrin) indirectly | from methylene blue (Fig. 1.2). Suramin, introduced in 1920, is a colourless compound having a useful action against human trypanosomiasis. Its particular value lies in its safety. It was the first useful antimicrobial drug without a toxic metal atom and the ratio of the dose required to produce toxic symptoms to that needed for a curative effect is vastly higher than with any of the arsenicals. It is also remarkably persistent, a single dose giving protection for more than a month. Mepacrine, first marketed in 1933, was an antimalarial agent of immense value in the Second

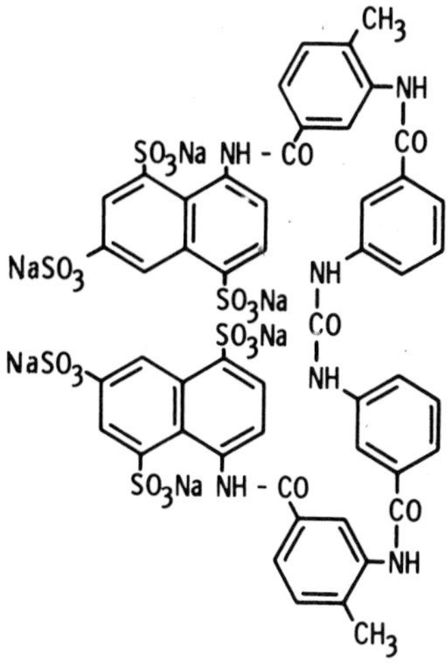

Figure 1.2 Early synthetic compounds used for treating diseases due to protozoa: suramin for trypanosomiasis (sleeping sickness) and mepacrine for malaria.

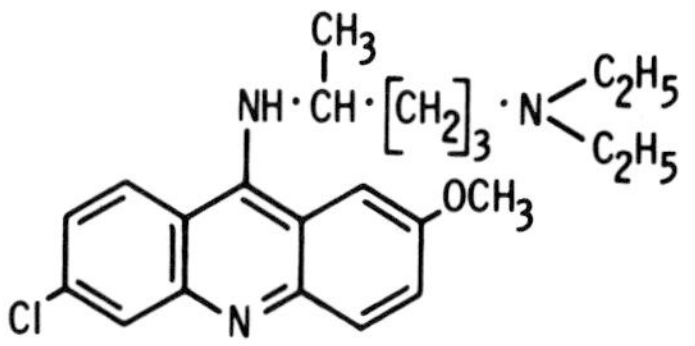

World War. It has been supplanted by other compounds partly because it causes a yellow discolouration of the skin. Besides these obvious descendants from Ehrlich's work the whole field of drug therapy is permeated by his ideas and many other important compounds can be traced directly or indirectly to the influence of his thought.

The treatment of bacterial infections by synthetic compounds

In spite of the successes achieved in the treatment of diseases caused by protozoa, the therapy of bacterial infections remained for many years an elusive and apparently unattainable goal. Ehrlich himself, in collaboration with Bechtold, made a series of phenols which showed much higher antibacterial potency than the simple phenols originally used as disinfectants. These compounds, however, had no effect on bacterial infections in animals. Other attempts were equally unsuccessful and no practical progress was made until 1935, when Domagk reported the activity of Prontosil rubrum against infections in animals. The discovery occurred in the course of a widespread research programme on the therapeutic use of dyestuffs, apparently inspired by Ehrlich's ideas. Tréfouël showed Prontosil rubrum to be broken down in the body giving sulphanilamide which was in fact the effective antibacterial agent. The story of this work and its

consequences are told in Chapter 6. The sulphonamides were out-
standingly successful drugs. They might have been developed and
used even more widely if penicillin and other antibiotics had not
followed on so speedily. Surprisingly in the field of synthetic antibacterial agents few other successes have been achieved against the
common bacterial infections. In part this may be due to the
diminished incentive to search for new products when the antibiotics
have proved to give such excellent results. However, synthetic
compounds with a useful action against bacterial infections have
certainly been extremely difficult to find. The only widely used
synthetic compounds apart from the sulphonamides are nalidixic
acid (Chapter 4), the nitrofuran antibacterials and trimethoprim
(Chapter 6). In contrast with most common bacterial infections,
those caused by the mycobacteria are usually more effectively treated
with synthetic agents than with antibiotics. For many years after
treatment was available for streptococcal and staphylococcal
infections, tuberculosis and leprosy remained untreatable by chemotherapy. The first success came with the antibiotic streptomycin,
which remains part of the standard treatment for tuberculosis. Very
soon afterwards however a number of chemically unrelated synthetic
agents were found to be effective against this disease. The best of
these are isonicotinic hydrazide and *p*-aminosalicylic acid (Chapter 6)
though several other types remain as second-line drugs. Apart from
streptomycin and its relatives the antibiotics have played relatively
little part in the treatment of tuberculosis. In leprosy the drug
regularly used is a synthetic compound, 4,4'-diaminodiphenyl-
sulphone.

The antibiotic revolution

Ever since bacteria have been cultivated on solid media contaminant
organisms have occasionally appeared on the plates. Sometimes this
foreign colony would be surrounded by an area in which bacterial
growth was suppressed. Usually this was regarded as a mere technical
nuisance, but Fleming, observing such an effect with a mould
Penicillium notatum on a plate seeded with staphylococci, was
struck by its potential importance. He showed that the mould
produced a freely diffusible substance highly active against Gram-
positive bacteria, and apparently of low toxicity to animals. He
named it penicillin. It was however unstable and early attempts to
extract it failed, so Fleming's observation lay neglected until 1939.
By then the success of the sulphonamides had stimulated a renewed
interest in the chemotherapy of bacterial infections. The search for

other antibacterial agents now seemed a promising and exciting project and Florey and Chain selected Fleming's penicillin for re-examination. They succeeded in isolating an impure but highly active solid preparation and published their results in 1940. Evidence of its great clinical usefulness in man followed in 1941. It was now apparent that a compound of revolutionary importance in medicine had been discovered. To make it generally available for medical use, however, presented formidable problems both in research and in large scale production, especially under conditions of war-time stringency. Eventually perhaps the biggest chemical and biological joint research programme ever mounted was undertaken, involving 39 laboratories in Britain and the United States. It was an untidy operation with much duplication and overlapping of work, but it culminated in the isolation of pure penicillin, the determination of its structure and the establishment of methods for its production on a large scale. The obstacles overcome in this research were enormous. They arose mainly from the very low concentrations of penicillin in the original mould cultures and from the marked chemical instability of the product. In the course of this work the concentration of penicillin in mould culture fluids was increased 1000-fold by the isolation of improved variants of *P. notatum* using selection and mutation methods and by improved conditions of culture. This tremendous improvement in yield was decisive in making large scale production practicable and ultimately cheap.

The success of penicillin quickly diverted a great deal of scientific effort towards the search for other antibiotics. The most prominent name in this development was that of Waksman who began an intensive search for antibiotics in moulds isolated from soil samples obtained from all parts of the world. Waksman's first success was streptomycin and many other antibiotics followed. Waksman's screening methods were copied in many other laboratories. Organisms of all kinds were examined and hundreds of thousands of cultures were tested. Further successes came quickly. Out of all this research some 3000 named antibiotics have been listed. Most of them, however, have defects that prevent their development as drugs. Perhaps 50 have had some sort of clinical use and many fewer are regularly employed in the therapy of infectious disease. However, among this select group are compounds of such excellent qualities that treatment is now available for almost all the bacterial and fungal infections known to occur in man. All this was achieved in the space of a mere twenty years.

New antibiotics continue to appear, but mostly these are variants of known types, without sufficient advantage to favour their use in place of well established compounds.

The most significant development of recent years has been the use of chemical modification to extend and improve the action of naturally occurring antibiotics. This was first done successfully with the penicillins (Chapter 2) and has since been extended to several other classes of antibiotics. The current development of antibiotics has swung away from the search for novel types. Instead research concentrates on taking antibiotics of known excellence and tailoring them to produce compounds with some special advantage, such as immunity to attack by bacterial enzymes. ✻

The synthetic antibacterials and the antibiotics illustrate a phenomenon that is not uncommon in the development of science. Sulphanilamide, isonicotinic hydrazide and *p*-aminosalicylic acid were all compounds known to chemistry long before their antibacterial potency was realized. Many of the antibiotics are produced by commonly occurring micro-organisms and are relatively easy to isolate. There is no technical reason why they should not have been found many years earlier. It required the stimulus of the chance discovery of the activity of the sulphonamides to encourage the large scale search that in fifteen years transformed the medical treatment of bacterial infection.

Reasons for studying the biochemistry of antimicrobial compounds

✻Following this brief survey of the discovery of the present wide range of antimicrobial compounds, we may now turn to the main theme of the book. We shall be concerned with the biochemical mechanisms that underlie the action of compounds used in the battle against micro-organisms. This topic has a twofold interest. In the long run a detailed understanding of antibacterial action at the molecular level may generate ideas for the design of entirely novel antimicrobial agents. In spite of the great power and success of the drugs currently available, there are still areas where improvements can undoubtedly be made. The other interest in antimicrobial agents is the light that their activity can throw on the subject of biochemistry itself. Antibacterial agents, particularly the antibiotics, often have a highly selective action on biochemical processes. They may block a single reaction within a complex sequence of events. The use of such agents has often revealed details of biochemical processes that would otherwise have been difficult to disentangle. Our present knowledge owes much to experiments with such compounds as puromycin, penicillin and oligomycin. Understanding of the biochemistry of antimicrobial action has been built up slowly and painfully with many false starts and setbacks. Since about 1960, however, a much greater insight into the action of antibacterial compounds has been achieved, and for most of the compounds commonly used in medical practice at least an outline can be given of the biochemical effects underlying their action on bacteria. In contrast, knowledge of the mechanism of action of antiprotozoal drugs, which were discovered long before the antibacterial drugs, has lagged well behind. This is due mainly to the much greater difficulty in isolating and working with protozoa outside the animal body, but interest has also been concentrated on bacteria because of their special importance in infectious disease and because of their widespread use in biochemical and genetic research.

Development of biochemical knowledge of antimicrobial action

Understanding of how antimicrobial compounds bring about their effects has accumulated gradually. Several levels of progress can be distinguished and will be separately discussed.

Pharmacological biochemistry

When an antimicrobial agent is used systemically its effectiveness is determined by various factors that govern its behaviour in the body. Means can usually be found for studying the absorption, distribution and excretion of the compound. Activity requires the maintenance of a sufficient concentration of the drug at the site of action; this concentration must continue long enough to allow the body's defences time to defeat the infection. The concentration attained depends on relative rates of absorption and excretion. It is also affected by metabolic changes brought about by the body's enzymes acting on the drug. Metabolism usually inactivates the antimicrobial agent, but several examples are known where metabolism is essential for converting an inactive administered compound into an active drug circulating in the body (Chapter 6). The degree of binding of the drug to various tissues may also be important. Some drugs are firmly bound to plasma proteins. This increases their persistence in the body but may also lower their effectiveness if activity depends on the concentration of free (unbound) compound present in the blood. There is always an equilibrium between free and bound drug but for strongly bound compounds the amount of drug in free solution may be very small. The methods for studying such factors are now well-established; it is often convenient to use drugs which carry a radioactive atom as a 'label' at some point in their molecule.

Information of this sort is a preliminary to understanding anti-microbial action. It can help to explain differences of effects between different species and for a new compound it gives a firm base for recommendations on the size and frequency of doses used in treating human patients.

Nature of the biochemical systems affected

As long as antimicrobial compounds have been known, workers have attempted to explain their action in biochemical terms. Ehrlich made a tentative beginning in this direction when he suggested that the arsenicals might act by combining with thiol groups on the protozoal cells. He was, however, severely limited by the elementary state of biochemistry at that period. By the time the sulphonamides were discovered the biochemistry of small molecules was much more advanced and reasonable biochemical explanations of sulphonamide action were soon available. However, many of the antibiotics which followed presented very different problems. Attempts to apply biochemical methods to the study of their action led to highly conflicting answers. At one stage a count showed that 14 different biochemical systems had been suggested as the site of action of streptomycin against bacteria. Much of this confusion arose from a failure to distinguish between primary and secondary effects. The biochemical processes of bacterial cells are closely interlinked. Hence disturbance of any one important system is likely to have effects on many of the others. Methods had to be developed that would distinguish between the primary biochemical effect of an anti-microbial agent and other changes in metabolism that followed as a consequence. Once these were established more accurate assessments could be made of the real site of action of various antimicrobial compounds. The limiting factor then became the extent of bio-chemical information about the nature of the target site. From about 1955 onwards there has been a dramatic increase in the understanding of the structure, function and synthesis of macromolecules. Most of the important antibiotics were found to act by interfering with the biosynthesis or function of macromolecules and the development of new techniques has provided the means of locating their site of action with some confidence.

Methods used for the study of the mode of action of antimicrobial compounds

Experience gained over the last fifteen years has helped to evolve reasonably systematic procedures for working out the primary sites of action of many antimicrobial compounds. Once the primary site of action is established the overall effect of a drug on the metabolism of microbial cells can often be explained. Many of the techniques used in elucidating the mode of action of antimicrobial agents are discussed in later chapters but it may be helpful to set them out in a logical sequence.

(1) Where the chemical structure is known, it is studied carefully to determine whether a structural analogy exists with part or whole of a biologically important molecule, i.e. a metabolic intermediate or essential cofactor, nutrient etc. An analogy may be immediately obvious, but sometimes it becomes apparent only through imaginative model building or by hindsight when the target site of the compound has been revealed by other means. Analogies of structure can sometimes be misleading and should only be used as a preliminary indication.

(2) The next step is to examine the effects of the compound on the growth kinetics and morphology of suitable bacteria. A cytocidal effect shown by reduction in viable count probably indicates damage to the cell membrane. This can be confirmed by observation of leakage of potassium ions, nucleotides or amino acids from the cells. Severe damage leads to cell lysis. Examination of cells by electron microscopy may show morphological changes which indicate interference with the synthesis of one of the components of the cell wall. Many antibiotics have only a cytostatic action and do not cause any detectable morphological changes.

(3) If the antimicrobial agent does not act by damaging the membrane, attempts are made to reverse its action by addition to the medium of various supplements. Nutrients including oxidizable carbon sources, fatty and amino acids, intermediary metabolites such as purines and pyrimidines, vitamins and bacterial growth factors are tested in turn. If reversal is achieved, this may point directly to the reaction or reaction sequence which is blocked by the inhibitor. Valuable confirmatory evidence can sometimes be obtained by the use of auxotrophic organisms requiring a compound known to be the next intermediate in a biosynthetic sequence beyond the reaction blocked by the antimicrobial agent. An auxotroph of this type should be resistant to the action of the inhibitor. Inhibition in a biosynthetic sequence may also be revealed by accumulation of the metabolite immediately *before* the blocked reaction. Unfortunately the actions of many antimicrobial agents are not reversed by exogenous compounds. This especially applies to compounds which interfere with the polymerization stages in nucleic acid and protein biosynthesis where reversal is impossible.

(4) The ability of an inhibitor to interfere with the supply and consumption of ATP is usually examined since any disturbance of energy metabolism has profound effects on the biological activity of the cell. The inhibitor is tested against the respiratory and glycolytic activies of the micro-organism, and the ATP content of the cells is measured.

(5) Useful information can often be gained by observing the effect of an antimicrobial agent on the kinetics of uptake of a radio-labelled nutrient, such as glucose, acetate, a fatty acid, an amino acid, phosphate etc. It is preferable to choose conditions where a steady uptake of nutrient is established. Changes in rate of incorporation which follow the addition of the drug are measured and compared with effects on growth. A prompt interference with incorporation of a particular nutrient may provide a good clue to the primary site of action.

(6) An antimicrobial compound that inhibits protein or nucleic acid synthesis in cells without interfering with (*i*) membrane functions, (*ii*) the biosynthesis of the immediate precursors of proteins and nucleic acids or (*iii*) the generation and utilization of ATP, very probably inhibits macromolecular synthesis at the polymerization level. Because of the close interrelationship between protein and nucleic acid synthesis indirect effects of the inhibition of one process on the other are carefully distinguished. For example, a compound that interferes directly with the biosynthesis of RNA indirectly inhibits protein biosynthesis as the supply of messenger RNA is exhausted. Again, inhibitors of protein synthesis eventually arrest DNA synthesis because of the requirement for continued protein biosynthesis for the initiation of new cycles of DNA replication (Chapter 5). A study of the kinetics of the inhibition of each macromolecular biosynthesis in intact cells is valuable since indirect inhibitions appear later than direct effects.

(7) When the inhibited biochemical system has been identified in intact cells, more detailed information can then be obtained with cell-free preparations. This may involve the isolation of suspected target enzymes, or cell organelles such as membranes, ribosomes or purified highly polymerized nucleic acids. The antimicrobial compound is tested for inhibitory activity against the suspected target reaction *in vitro*. In this way more insight may be gained about the molecular nature of the interaction between the inhibitor and the target site. There is always a danger, however, of non-specific effects *in vitro* especially at high concentrations of drug. Failure to inhibit the suspected target reaction *in vitro* on the other hand even with very high concentrations of drug cannot rule out inhibition of the

same reaction in intact cells for a number of reasons: (*i*) The drug may be metabolized either by the host or by the micro-organism to an inhibitory derivative. (*ii*) Extensive purification of an enzyme may desensitize it to the inhibitor by altering an allosteric target. (*iii*) The site of inhibition in the intact cell may be part of a highly integrated structural assembly which is disrupted during the preparation of a cell-free system again causing a loss of sensitivity to the inhibitor. The use of cell-free preparations from drug-resistant mutants is sometimes useful in the exact localization of the point of attack. This approach has been ingeniously exploited in identifying the target site of streptomycin in bacterial ribosomes (Chapter 4).

Mode of action studies should not be undertaken lightly. They may involve a considerable research effort, and success cannot be guaranteed. There are still a number of well-known antimicrobials for which no completely satisfactory answer concerning their primary biochemical target has been forthcoming.

Selectivity of action of antimicrobial agents

In the study of any useful antimicrobial agent it is not sufficient just to explain its action on the metabolism of the micro-organism. The compound must by definition be selective in its action, and a reason must be sought for this selectivity. Thus it is usually necessary to study the actions of these compounds on the biochemistry of the host cell as well as that of the parasite. The basis of selectivity varies from one drug to another. The process inhibited may occur only in the microbial cell, so there is no reason for the host cells to be affected. Other agents act on biochemical mechanisms found in both microbial and animal cells, but for some reason affect only the former. In such cases the reason for this differential action is still obscure and evidently requires further study. Yet another type of selectivity depends on the concentrating of the antimicrobial agent within the microbial cell, but not in the host cell. Thus even though at the ultimate site of action the drug is equally inhibitory to both, its greater concentration in the micro-organism ensures the necessary selectivity. Here the question shifts to the reason for the selective concentration, and our knowledge of these mechanisms is still scanty.

The molecular interaction between the antimicrobial agent and the target site

The objective of a mode of action study on an antimicrobial agent is to relate its biological effects on sensitive cells to the interaction between the inhibitor and its biochemical target in the cells. Ultimately this requires the interaction to be explained in molecular terms. Not only therefore do we need to understand the chemical structure and properties of the inhibitor molecule in great detail but we need similarly detailed knowledge of the target site. At present this is where almost all mode of action models stop, as we simply do not have enough information about the target sites. The reason for this is clear enough: all inhibitor targets are macromolecules and despite considerable advances in molecular biology the study of most of these targets in chemical terms is in its infancy. Not until this challenge is met shall we be able to account for the essential chemical features of most antimicrobial drugs or make much progress towards the rational design of new or improved agents.

Meanwhile a start may be made by studying the exact structural requirements for antimicrobial activity. With the complex antibiotics the structures of active molecules are highly specific; minor chemical changes can result in complete inactivation. Only with a few quite simple compounds can the significance of chemical structure be satisfactorily explained in terms of biological activity. A successful antimicrobial suitable for systemic use must have a combination of properties: suitable absorption and distribution in the animal body, ability to penetrate or concentrate in the micro-organism, and selective action on a target site within the cell. Each of these may require some different molecular feature. For optimum activity all these features must be present together in the same molecule and must not interfere with one another. The success of the best antibiotics may be due to contributions by different parts of the molecule to the overall pattern of action. Biochemical research on isolated systems may eventually distinguish the contributions of these different components.

The biochemistry of microbial resistance

The therapeutic value of an antimicrobial agent often declines after prolonged use through the emergence of organisms which are no longer sensitive to the compound. This problem of expanding practical importance has been studied by microbiological and biochemical methods. Such studies will usually show the means by which resistance has been acquired, either by selection or by genetic-transfer through an R-factor or by phage infection. They will also define the biochemical changes that render an organism resistant. The results of such studies are discussed in Chapter 8. The mechanism of some forms of resistance still needs further study and there is obviously great practical interest in methods of preventing the acquisition of resistance or of combating resistance once it has arisen.

The practical value of resistance studies has already been proved by the development of successful antibacterials in which the original molecules have been chemically modified to render them insusceptible to bacterial enzymes responsible for important types of resistance.

Scope and layout of the present book

In this book we have tried to select well-established evidence for the biochemical action of nearly all the best-known antibacterial and antifungal agents used in medicine. Those compounds where the mode of action is in considerable doubt receive only passing mention. Some antimicrobial compounds of particular biochemical significance are also included even though they have no therapeutic value. A short section brings together information on the action of antifungal agents including some which are used against plant pathogens. Compounds active against protozoa are discussed, though many important compounds are left unmentioned because of the lack of information on their biochemical action. The few compounds showing activity against human virus infections are dealt with briefly.

Antibacterial and antifungal compounds have been classified according to their type of biochemical action rather than on grounds of chemical structure. The last two chapters consider the mechanisms by which antimicrobial compounds enter the target cells, and the biochemistry of the development of resistance to antibacterial agents.

Further reading

General works on antimicrobial compounds and their action

Books

E.F. GALE, E. CUNDLIFFE, P.E. REYNOLDS, M.H. RICHMOND and M.J. WARING (1972), *The Molecular Basis of Antibiotic Action* (John Wiley & Sons, 1972).

W.B. PRATT (1973), *Fundamentals of Chemotherapy* (Oxford University Press, 1973).

L.P. GARROD, H.P. LAMBERT and F. O'GRADY (1973), *Antibiotic and Chemotherapy*, 4th edn. (Churchill Livingstone, 1973).

D. GOTTLIEB and P.D. SHAW (eds) (1967), *Antibiotics*, Vol. 1, Mechanism of Action (Springer Verlag, 1967).

J.W. CORCORAN and F.E. HAHN (eds) (1975), *Antibiotics*, Vol. 3, Mechanism of Action of Antimicrobial and Antitumour Agents (Springer Verlag, 1975).

F.E. HAHN (ed) (1979), *Antibiotics*, Vol. 5, Part 1, Mechanism of Action of Antibacterial Agents; Part 2, Mechanism of Action of Antieukaryotic and

Antiviral Compounds (Springer Verlag, 1979).

W.B. HUGO and A.D. RUSSELL (eds) (1977), *Pharmaceutical Microbiology* (Blackwell, 1977).

HAMAO UMEZAWA (ed), *Index of Antibiotics from Actinomycetes*, Vol. 1, 1967, Vol. 2, 1978 (Japanese Scientific Societies Press).

J.S. GLASBY (1979), *Encyclopaedia of Antibiotics*, 2nd edn. (Wiley, 1979).

H. SENECA (1971), *Biological Basis of Chemotherapy of Infections and Infestations* (F.A. Davis & Co., 1971).

A. GOLDSTEIN, L. ARONOW and S.M. KALMAN (1974), *Principles of Drug Action*, 2nd edn. (Wiley International, 1974).

T. KORZYBSKI, Z. KOWSZYK-GINDIFER and W. KURYLOWICZ (1979), *Antibiotics, Origin, Nature and Properties* (3 vols.), English edn. (American Society for Microbiology, 1979).

Review articles

A.P. BALL and A.M. GEDDES (1979), 'New antibiotics - a review' in *Recent Adv. Infect.*, 1, 19.

J. BÉRDY (1974), 'Classification of antibiotics by chemical structure' in *Adv. Appl. Microbiol.*, 18, 309.

S.S. COHEN (1979), 'Comparative biochemistry and drug design for infectious disease' in *Science*, 205, 964.

A.P. BALL, J.A. GRAY and J.McC. MURDOCH (1975), 'Antibacterial drugs today' Parts 1 and 2 in *Drugs*, 10, 1 and 81.

H. ZÄHNER (1977), 'Some aspects of antibiotic research' in *Angew. Chem. Int. Ed.*, 16, 687.

2 The bacterial cell wall – a vulnerable shield

Functions of the wall

In the search for differences between bacteria and animal cells that could provide the basis for a selective antibacterial attack, one evident distinction lies in their general structure. The animal cell is relatively large and has a complex organization; its biochemical processes are compartmentalized and different functions are served by the nucleus with its surrounding membrane, by the mitochondria and by various other organelles. The outer membrane is thin and lacks rigidity. The cell exists in an environment controlled in temperature and in osmolarity and it is constantly supplied with nutrients from the extracellular fluid bathing it. The smaller bacterial cell lives in a variable, and often unfavourable environment. In particular it must be able to withstand considerable changes in osmolarity. Some bacteria have relatively high concentrations of solutes of low molecular weight in their cytoplasm. Such a cell suspended in water or in dilute solutions will develop a high internal osmotic pressure. This would inevitably disrupt its membrane unless it were provided with a tough, rigid outer coat. This coat is the cell wall, a characteristic bacterial structure entirely lacking in animal cells. It has a protective function for the bacterium, but at the same time it is vulnerable to attack, and a number of effective antibacterials owe their action to their ability to disturb the processes by which the wall is synthesized. Since there is no parallel biosynthetic mechanism in the animal cell, substances affecting this process may have quite a low toxicity.

The term 'wall' will be used to describe all the cell covering which lies outside the cytoplasmic membrane. 'Envelope' comprises both the wall and the cytoplasmic membrane.

Wall structure

Bacterial wall structure varies considerably from one species to another, but follows general patterns which are related to the broad morphological classification of bacteria. Classically this has been based on behaviour towards the Gram stain, but the well-tried division into Gram-positive and Gram-negative types has a significance far beyond that of an empirical staining reaction. The most evident differences are worth recalling.

Many Gram-negative bacteria are highly adaptable organisms which will use inorganic nitrogen compounds, mineral salts and a simple carbon source for synthesis of their whole structure. Their cytoplasm has a relatively low osmolarity. The typical Gram-positive coccus or bacillus tends to be more exacting in its nutritional needs. Such organisms lack some synthetic abilities and require various amino acids, vitamins and accessory factors for growth. They are usually cultivated on rich, undefined broths or on fairly elaborate synthetic media. They concentrate amino acids, nucleotides and other metabolites of low molecular weight in their cytoplasm and consequently have a high internal osmolarity. Bacteria do not all fit this neat division. The Gram-negative cocci, the rickettsias, the chlamydias and the spirochetes, for example, are all Gram-negative bacteria with exacting growth requirements. The mycoplasmas lack a rigid wall structure and, although technically Gram-negative, are best treated as a separate group lying outside the usual Gram stain classification.

Most of the work on wall structure has been done with Gram-positive cocci and bacilli and with enteric bacteria and other Gram-negative rods. The extent to which the structural generalizations apply to groups outside these classes is uncertain.

The Gram-positive wall

Many Gram-positive bacteria have relatively simple walls. The wall, which lies above the cell membrane, is usually between 15 and 50 nm thick. For biochemical studies, bacteria are broken by shaking a suspension with small glass beads; the walls are separated from cytoplasmic material by washing and differential centrifugation. In electron micrographs these wall preparations resemble empty envelopes, torn in places where the cytoplasmic contents were released. With Gram-positive bacteria the wall is obtained relatively free from other bacterial components, but Gram-negative wall preparations (Fig. 2.1) usually contain some material from the cytoplasmic membrane.

The major part of the Gram-positive wall is a large polymer comprising two covalently linked components. One of these

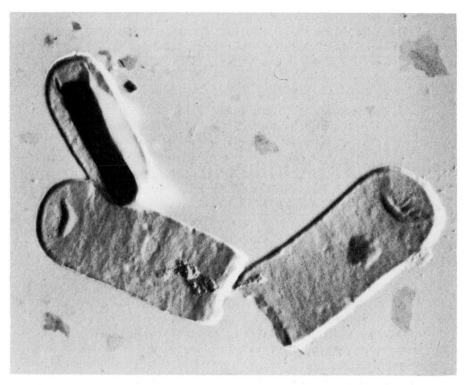

Figure 2.1 Electron micrograph of isolated cell envelopes from *Pseudomonas aeruginosa* shadowed with metal. We thank Mr A. Davies and Mrs M. Bentley for this picture.

components, forming at least 50 of the wall mass, is peptidoglycan (sometimes referred to as murein or mucopeptide). Its cross-linked structure provides a tough, fibrous fabric giving strength and shape to the cell and enabling it to withstand a high internal osmotic pressure. The amount of peptidoglycan in the wall shows that it covers the cell in a multi-layered structure, with cross-linking both within and between the layers. Attached to the peptidoglycan is an acidic polymer, accounting for 30-40 of the wall mass, which differs from species to species. Often this is a teichoic acid — a substituted poly (D-ribitol-5-phosphate) (see Fig. 2.7) — or a substituted glycerol-3-phosphate. In some bacteria teichoic acid is replaced by poly(*N*-acetylglucosamine-l-phosphate) or teichuronic acid (a polymer containing uronic acid and *N*-acetylhexosamine units). Bacteria that normally incorporate teichoic acid in their walls can switch to teichuronic acid under conditions of phosphate limitation. The acidic character of the polymer attached to the peptidoglycan ensures that the cell surface is strongly polar and carries a negative charge. This may influence the passage of ions, particulary Mg^{2+}, into the cell.

The teichoic acid or other acidic polymer is readily solubilized and released from the insoluble peptidoglycan by hydrolysis in cold acid or alkali. The nature of the linkage is described later.

Other components of the Gram-positive wall vary widely from species to species. Protein is often present to the extent of 5 to 10 per cent, and protein A of *Staphylococcus aureus* is apparently linked covalently to peptidoglycan. Proteins and polysaccharides frequently occur in the outermost layers and provide the main source of the antigenic properties of these bacteria. Mycobacteria and a few related genera differ from other Gram-positive bacteria in having large amounts of complex lipids in their wall structure.

The Gram-negative wall

The Gram-negative wall is far more complex. Wide-ranging studies of its structure have been concentrated on the enterobacteriaceae and on *Escherichia coli* in particular.

When cells of *E.coli* are fixed, stained with suitable metal salts, sectioned and examined by electron microscopy, the cytoplasmic membrane can be readily identified by its usual 'sandwich' appearance of two electron-dense layers separated by a lighter space. Above this, the cell wall appears as a structure containing three electron-dense layers separated by clear layers (Fig. 2.2). The clear layer immediately outside the cytoplasmic membrane is described as the periplasmic space. Here are found soluble enzymes and other components which can be released by submitting the cell to transient, non-lethal osmotic shock. The electron-dense layer, about 2 nm thick, immediately outside the periplasmic space represents the peptidoglycan component of the wall. It is much thinner than in Gram-positive bacteria and may constitute only 5 per cent or less of the wall mass. Even so it contributes substantially to wall strength. Cells rapidly lyse when treated with lysozyme, an enzyme which specifically degrades peptidoglycan. In *E.coli* the peptidoglycan is covalently linked to a lipoprotein which probably projects into the outer regions of the wall. The outer regions of the Gram-negative cell wall have been the most difficult to characterize. The various components together form a structure 6-10 nm thick, called the outer membrane. Like the cytoplasmic membrane it is basically a lipid bilayer, hydrophobic in the interior with hydrophilic groups at the outer surfaces. It also has protein components which penetrate the layer partly or completely

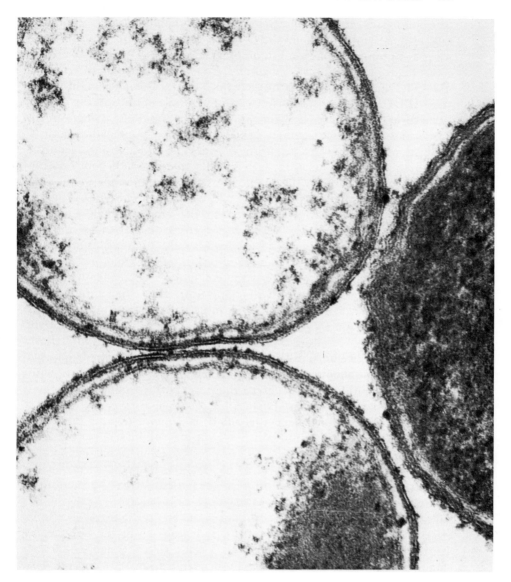

Figure 2.2 Electron micrograph of cross-section of parts of *E.coli* cells showing the multiple structure of cell wall and cell membrane. We thank Mr A. Davies and Mrs M. Bentley for this picture.

and form the membrane 'mosaic'. Despite these broad structural similarities, the outer membrane differs widely in composition and function from the cytoplasmic membrane. Its main constitutents are lipopolysaccharide, phospholipids, fatty acids and proteins. The phospholipids, mainly phosphatidyl ethanolamine and phosphatidyl glycerol, resemble those in the cytoplasmic membrane. The structure of the lipopolysaccharide is complex and varies considerably from one bacterial strain to another. The molecule has three parts (see Fig. 2.3). The core is built from 3-deoxy-D-*manno*-octulosonic acid (KDO), hexoses, heptoses, ethanolamine and phosphoric acid as structural components. The three KDO residues contribute a structural unit which strongly binds the divalent ions of magnesium and calcium, an important feature stabilizing the membrane. Removal of these ions by chelating agents leads to release of some of the lipopolysaccharide into the medium; at the same time the membrane becomes permeable to compounds that would otherwise be excluded. The core polysaccharide is linked to the antigenic side chain, a polysaccharide which can vary greatly from one strain to another even within the same bacterial species. Usually it comprises about 30 sugar units, although these can vary both in number and in structure. It forms the outermost layer of the cell and is the main source of its antigenic characteristics. At the opposite end, the core of the lipopolysaccharide is attached to a moiety known as lipid A which can be hydrolysed to glucosamine, long-chain fatty acids, phosphate and ethanolamine. The fatty acid chains of lipid A, along with those of the phospholipids, align themselves to form the hydrophobic interior of the membrane. The outer membrane is asymmetric with lipopolysaccharide exclusively on the outer surface and phospholipid mainly on the inner surface.

Many proteins have been identified as components of the outer membrane. The most abundant in *E.coli* are the matrix protein and lipoprotein. Matrix protein, also known as protein 1, has been fully sequenced. Its molecular weight is 37 205. Together with other rather similar proteins it forms a hexagonal lattice in the outer membrane with a 7.7 nm repeating unit. This pattern is best seen by electron microscopy of spheroplasts lacking peptidoglycan. Such examination also reveals triplets of indentations in the membrane surface each 2 nm in diameter, and 3 nm apart, through which the stain used in the preparation readily penetrates. This is interpreted as showing that the matrix protein molecules stretch across the membrane in groups of three, enclosing pores through which water and small molecules can pass. Such proteins have therefore been called porins. The size of the pores explains the selective permeability of the bacterial wall, allowing the entry of hydrophilic molecules up to a maximum molecular weight of 600 to 700. Artificial vesicles can be made with outer membrane lipids. Without protein these are impermeable to solutes, but when porins are incorporated they show

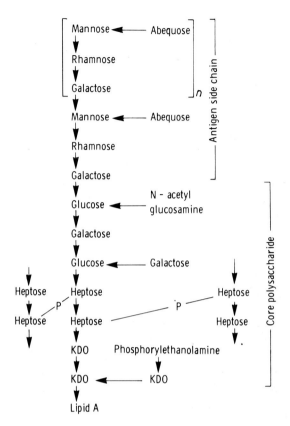

Figure 2.3 Tentative structure of the lipopolysaccharide of the cell envelope of *S. typhimurium*. The diagram has been simplified by omitting the configuration of the glycosidic linkages and omitting the *O*-acetyl groups from the abequose units. KDO: 3-deoxy-D-*manno*octulosonic acid. Lipid A consists of a β-1, 6-linked diglucosamine residue to which lauric, myristic, palmitic and 3-D(-) hydroxymyristic acids are bound. The heptose residues of three lipopolysaccharide polymers are shown linked by phosphate diester bridges although an alternative view is that the polymers may be interlinked by pyrophosphate bridges between the diglucosamine residues of lipid A. Although there are considerable structural variations in the antigen side chain among *Salmonella* species, the core poly-saccharide and lipid A are probably common to all wild-type *Salmonellae*. The core structure in *E.coli* is more variable.

permeability characteristics similar to those of the outer membrane itself.

Lipoprotein is another major component of the outer membrane proteins. About one-third is linked to peptidoglycan and the remaining two-thirds is unattached, but forms part of the membrane. The nature of the attachment of lipoprotein to the side chains of peptidoglycan is discussed later. About one in twelve of the peptide side chains is thus substituted. The arrangement provides a structural anchorage of the outer membrane to the peptidoglycan layer. The fatty acid chains of the lipoprotein presumably align themselves in the hydrophobic inner layer of the outer membrane and the protein moiety may possibly associate with matrix protein, reinforcing the pore structure.

Many other proteins with specialized functions have been identified in the outer membrane. Some of these are transport proteins, allowing access to molecules such as vitamin B_{12} or nucleosides which are too large to penetrate the pores of the membrane. These proteins also possess receptor sites which are recognized by specific phages which attack the bacteria.

Structure and biosynthesis of peptidoglycan

The structure and biosynthesis of peptidoglycan have special significance relative to the action of a number of important antibacterials and have been studied extensively.

The biosynthesis of peptidoglycan was first worked out with *S. aureus*. Although bacteria show many variations in peptidoglycan structure, the biosynthetic sequence in *S. aureus* will serve to illustrate the general features of the process.

Cell walls from *S. aureus* were gently hydrolysed with trichloroacetic acid to remove the teichoic acid. The insoluble peptidoglycan was then hydrolysed with hot mineral acid. The hydrolysate contained amino sugars and the four amino acids, glycine, alanine, glutamic acid and lysine in the ratio 5:2:1:1. A clue to the structure and to the early stages of biosynthesis was an observation by Park that subinhibitory concentrations of penicillin caused the accumulation of three nucleotides. He determined their main features, and it is now known that these compounds were III (Fig. 2.4), IV (Fig. 2.5) and the intermediate between these two in which only L-alanine had been attached. The significance of these compounds was not recognized at the time, but later, when it became apparent that penicillin probably inhibits cell wall biosynthesis, the similarity between the hydrolysis products of peptidoglycan and of the Park nucleotides was evident. From this and other experiments the peptidoglycan structure was gradually pieced together and the details of its biosynthesis were worked out, mainly by Strominger and Tipper. The biosynthesis may be conveniently divided into four stages.

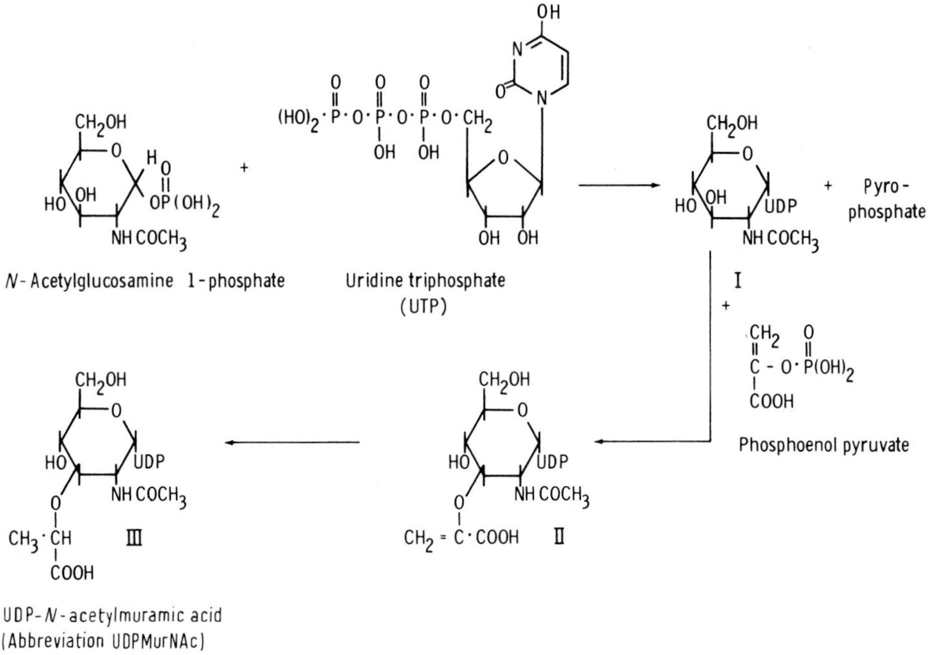

Figure 2.4 Peptidoglycan synthesis in *Staphylococcus aureus*. Stage 1: formation of UDP-*N*-acetylmuramic acid.

Stage 1. Synthesis of UDP-*N*-acetylmuramic acid

The biosynthesis starts with two products from the normal metabolic pool: *N*-acetylglucosamine-l-phosphate and UTP (Fig. 2.4). UDP-*N*-acetylglucosamine (I) is formed by the usual elimination of pyrophosphate. This nucleotide reacts with phosphoenolpyruvate by means of a specific transferase to give the corresponding 3-enolpyruvyl ether (II). The pyruvyl group is then converted to lactyl by a reductase requiring NADPH, the product being UDP-*N*-acetylmuramic acid (III, UDPMurNAc). Muramic acid (*3-0*-D-lactyl-D-glucosamine) is a distinctive amino sugar derivative found only in the peptidoglycan of cell walls.

Stage 2. Building the pentapeptide side chain

Five amino acid residues are next added to the carboxyl group of the muramic acid nucleotide (Fig. 2.5). Each step requires ATP and a specific enzyme. L-Alanine is added first. The next two residues are D-glutamic acid and then L-lysine. The lysine however is attached

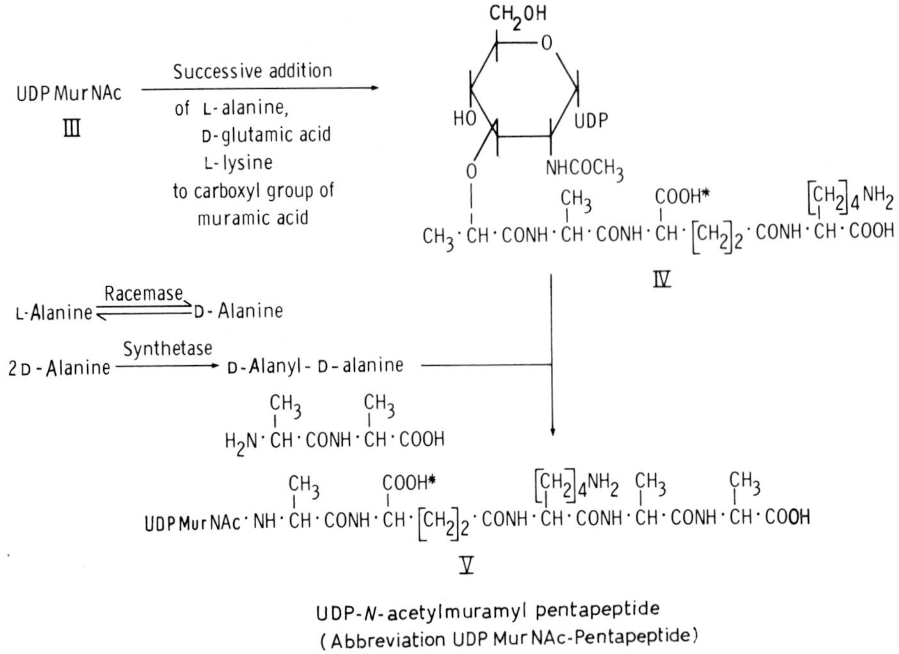

UDP Mur NAc
III
→ Successive addition
of L-alanine,
D-glutamic acid
L-lysine
to carboxyl group of
muramic acid

CH_2OH

HO

O

UDP

$NHCOCH_3$

CH_3 $COOH^*$ $[CH_2]_4NH_2$

$CH_3 \cdot CH \cdot CONH \cdot CH \cdot CONH \cdot CH \cdot [CH_2]_2 \cdot CONH \cdot CH \cdot COOH$

IV

L·Alanine $\overset{\text{Racemase}}{\rightleftharpoons}$ D·Alanine

2 D·Alanine $\overset{\text{Synthetase}}{\longrightarrow}$ D·Alanyl·D·alanine

CH_3 CH_3
$H_2N \cdot CH \cdot CONH \cdot CH \cdot COOH$

CH_3 $COOH^*$ $[CH_2]_4NH_2$ CH_3 CH_3
UDP MurNAc $\cdot$ NH $\cdot$ CH $\cdot$ CONH $\cdot$ CH $\cdot [CH_2]_2 \cdot$ CONH $\cdot$ CH $\cdot$ CONH $\cdot$ CH $\cdot$ CONH $\cdot$ CH $\cdot$ COOH

V

UDP-*N*-acetylmuramyl pentapeptide
(Abbreviation UDP Mur NAc-Pentapeptide)

Figure 2.5 Peptidoglycan synthesis. Stage 2: formation of UDP-*N*-acetylmuramyl pentapeptide. Addition of each amino acid and the final dipeptide requires ATP and a specific enzyme. L-Lysine is added to the γ-carboxyl group of D-glutamic acid; the α-carboxyl group (marked *) is amidated at a later stage in the biosynthesis.

through its α-amino group to the γ-carboxyl group of the glutamic acid. The α-carboxyl group of the glutamic acid is amidated at a later stage in the biosynthesis, so the second amino acid residue is sometimes referred to as D-*iso*glutamine. The biosynthesis of the pentapeptide is completed by addition not of an amino acid but of a dipeptide, D-alanyl-D-alanine, which is separately synthesized. A racemase acting on L-alanine gives D-alanine, and a synthetase then joins two molecules giving the dipeptide. The completed UDP-*N*-acetylmuramyl intermediate (V) with its pendant peptide group will be referred to as the 'nucleotide pentapeptide'.

Stage 3. Membrane-bound reactions leading to a linear peptidoglycan polymer

The biosynthesis up to this point involves relatively small molecules and the reactions are well characterized. The succeeding steps occur on membrane structures and are therefore less certainly defined. Although the course of each individual reaction is well established, the reaction sequence and the mode of attachment of newly synthesized units to existing wall material is still uncertain.

The first step involves the formation of a pyrophosphate link between the nucleotide pentapeptide and undecaprenyl phosphate (the phosphate ester of a C_{55} isoprenoid alcohol) which is a component of the cytoplasmic membrane (Fig. 2.6). In this reaction UMP is released and becomes available for reconversion to UTP which is needed in the first step of peptidoglycan biosynthesis (Fig. 2.4). All subsequent reactions occurring while the intermediates are linked to undecaprenyl phosphate take place without release from the membrane. An essential step in this membrane-bound reaction sequence is the addition of a second hexosamine residue through a typical glycosidation by UDP-N-acetylglucosamine (Fig. 2.6). The disaccharide (VII) is formed by a 1-4β linkage with liberation of UDP. The involvement of undecaprenyl phosphate is not unique to peptidoglycan biosynthesis. It is also concerned in the biosynthesis of the polysaccharide chain in the O-antigen produced by *Salmonella typhimurium* and in the formation of the polysaccharide elements of the lipopolysaccharides of Gram-negative bacteria; in Gram-positive bacteria it fulfils a similar role in the biosynthesis of teichoic acid or polysaccharides of the wall.

At about this point in the biosynthesis of *S. aureus* peptidoglycan an extending group is added to the ϵ-amino group of the lysine unit in the nucleotide pentapeptide. Glycine and a glycine-specific transfer RNA are involved in this process during which a pentaglycine group is added. The reaction, unlike the tRNA reactions in protein biosynthesis, does not require the presence of ribosomes; the five glycine units are added successively to the lysine from the nitrogen end (the reverse direction to protein biosynthesis). Since the resultant product (VIII) has 10 amino acid units it will be referred to as the disaccharide decapeptide. This still has a free terminal amino group. In the biosynthesis of peptidoglycans from certain other bacterial species no extending group is added. Later reactions then involve the ϵ-amino group of lysine (or equivalent diamino acid) instead of the terminal amino group of glycine. Also during the membrane-bound stage in the biosynthesis of *S. aureus* peptidoglycan the carboxyl group of D-glutamic acid is amidated by a reaction with ammonia and ATP. The exact sequence of these three reactions, addition of N-acetylglucosamine, chain extension and amidation is uncertain.

The final reaction in this stage is the attachment of the disaccharide decapeptide (VIII) to an undefined 'acceptor' present in the

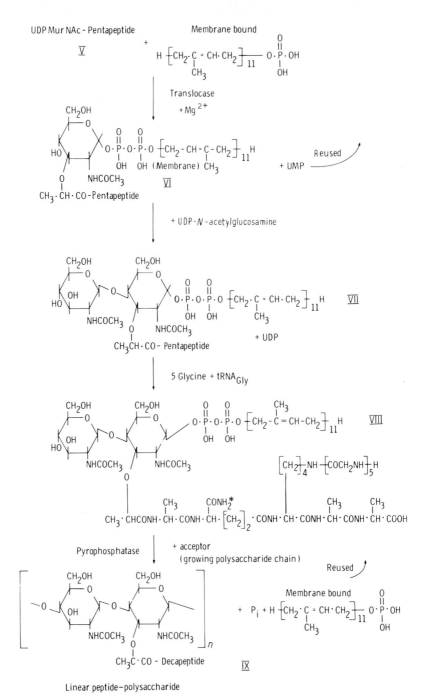

Figure 2.6 Peptidoglycan synthesis. Stage 3: formation of the linear peptidoglycan. The structure of the decapeptide side chain is shown in VIII; the point at which the amide group * is added has not yet been established.

particulate preparations that have been used for investigating these reactions. This acceptor is usually regarded as the growing linear polymer chain. In this reaction the disaccharide with its decapeptide side chain forms a β-linkage from the 1 position of the *N*-acetyl-muramic acid residue to the 4-hydroxyl group of the terminal *N*-acetylglucosamine residue in the growing polysaccharide chain. The membrane lipid is left as undecaprenyl pyrophosphate and is reconverted by a specific pyrophosphatase to the corresponding phosphate ready for another cycle of the membrane-bound part of the synthesis. The growth of the glycan chains thus occurs by successive addition of disaccharide units.

Stage 4. Cross-linking

The linear peptidoglycan (IX) formed in stage 3 contains many polar groups which make it soluble in water. It lacks rigidity and toughness. These attributes are introduced by cross-linking, a process well known in the plastic industry for producing similar results in synthetic linear polymers. The reactions leading to the linear peptidoglycan are intracellular or are intimately associated with the cytoplasmic membrane. The energy linked synthetic steps are brought about by conventional biochemical reactions. However, the final stage of peptidoglycan formation when the rigid, cross-linked structure is laid down, must take place outside the cell membrane, since the material once formed is insoluble and could not be moved from one site to another. The mechanism involved in cross-linking seems specially adapted to this situation; it is a transpeptidation reaction requiring no external supply of ATP or similar compounds. The transpeptidation occurs between the terminal amino group of the pentaglycine side chain and the peptide imino group of the terminal D-alanine residue of another peptide side chain; D-alanine is eliminated and a peptide bond is formed (Fig. 2.7). The loss of D-alanine in this reaction explains a feature that originally caused difficulty in under-standing the biosynthetic process. The ratio of alanine (D and L) to glutamic acid or to lysine in *S. aureus* peptidoglycan was well established as about 2:1, whilst in the 'pentapeptide' which was the apparent precursor the ratio was 3:1. The transpeptidation process explains this apparent anomaly. In *S. aureus* peptidoglycan the cross-linking is quite extensive and up to 10 peptide side chains may be bound together by bridging groups. Since the linear polymers them-selves are large it is possible that the whole of the peptidoglycan in a Gram-positive bacterium may be made up of units covalently bound together. This gigantic bag-shaped molecule has been called a

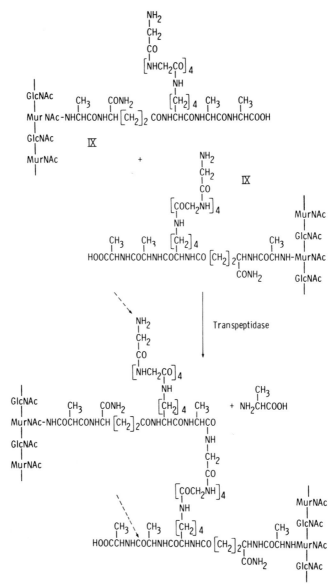

Figure 2.7 Peptidoglycan synthesis. Stage 4: cross-linking of two linear peptidoglycan chains. The linear polymers have the structure IX (Fig. 2.6) GlcNAc = *N*-acetylglucosaminyl residue. Broken arrows show points at which further cross-links may be formed with other polymer chains.

'sacculus'. However, even if this extensive covalent bonding really occurs there must be a mechanism for constantly breaking it down and reforming it to allow for cell growth and division. Enzymes which hydrolyse the polysaccharide chains and others attacking the peptide cross-links have been isolated from bacteria and probably exert this essential catabolic function during cell growth.

The cross-linking step has been difficult to study because the transpeptidases are found in particulate fractions from cell envelopes and no method has yet been found for releasing them without inactivation. Progress made with soluble extracellular enzymes and with low-molecular-weight substrates will be discussed later.

Variations in peptidoglycan structure

Many variations are found in peptidoglycan structure between one species of bacteria and another, or even between strains of the same species. Only a general account is possible here. Fuller details will be found in reviews listed at the end of the chapter. All peptidoglycans have the same glycan chain as in *S. aureus* except that the glucosamine residues are sometimes *N*-acylated with a group other than acetyl. The peptide side chains always have four amino acid units alternating L-, D-, L-, D- in configuration. The second residue is always D-glutamic acid, linked through its γ-carboxyl group, and the fourth always D-alanine. The peptidoglycan from *S. aureus*, classified by Strominger as Type A2, is characteristic of many cocci. Peptidoglycans of this group, and the related Types A3 and A4, have similar tetrapeptide side chains but vary in their bridging groups. The amino acids in the bridge are usually glycine, alanine, serine or threonine and the number of residues can vary from one to five. In Type A1 peptidoglycans the L-lysine of the Type II peptide side chain is usually replaced by *meso*-2,6-diaminopimelic acid, and there is no bridging group. Cross-linking occurs between the D-alanine of one side chain and the 6-amino group of the diaminopimelic acid of another. This peptidoglycan type is characteristic of many rod-shaped bacteria, both the large family of Gram-negative rods and the Gram-positive bacilli. In the less common Type B peptidoglycans cross-linkage occurs between the α-carboxyl group of the D-glutamic acid of one peptide side chain and the D-alanine of another, through a bridge containing a basic amino acid.

Cross-linking in Gram-negative bacteria

In contrast to the multiple random cross-linkage of peptidoglycan which is found in the Gram-positive cocci, the peptidoglycan of

E.coli and similar Gram-negative rods shows on average only a single cross-link between one peptide side chain and another. These bacteria contain, besides the transpeptidases concerned in cross-linkage, other enzymes known as DD-carboxypetidases which specifically remove D-alanine from a pentapeptide side chain. Carboxypeptidase I is specific for the terminal D-alanine of the pentapeptide side chain, whilst carboxypeptidase II acts on the D-alanine at position 4 after the terminal D-alanine has been removed. DD-Carboxypeptidase I seems in some way to limit the extent of cross-linking.

Growing evidence suggests that in *E.coli* the formation of peptidoglycan for wall extension differs in some way from that involved in septum production. Mirelman (1976) proposed that the nascent peptidoglycan used for wall extension acts as a carboxyl donor through its terminal D-alanyl-D-alanine sequences with the peptidoglycan in the wall providing the amino group acceptor. Other nascent peptidoglycan units are stripped of their terminal D-alanine by DD-carboxypeptidase I and accumulate at the equator of the cell. They then act as amino group acceptors for other peptidoglycan units retaining their D-alanyl-D-alanine terminus in cross-linking which provides new polymeric peptidoglycan to form the septum. The distinction between these processes is relevant to the action of β-lactam antibiotics (see below).

Attachments to peptidoglycans

Within the cell wall the polymeric peptidoglycan is usually only part of a larger polymer. In Gram-positive cocci it is linked to an acidic polymer, often a teichoic acid (Fig. 2.8).

The point of attachment is through the 6-hydroxyl group of muramic acid in the glycan chain. Only a small fraction of the muramic acid residues are thus substituted. In *S. aureus* cell walls teichoic acid is joined to peptidoglycan by a linking unit comprising three glycerol l-phosphate units attached to the 4-position of *N*-acetylglucosamine which engages through a phosphodiester group at position 1 with the 6-hydroxyl group of muramic acid. This type of linkage seems to occur with polymers other than teichoic acid, e.g. with poly(*N*-acetylglucosamine-1-phosphate) in a *Micrococcus* species. The acid-labile *N*-acetylglucosamine-1-phosphate linkage and the alkali-labile phosphodiester linkage at position 4 explain the ease with which teichoic acid can be split off from peptidoglycan. Within the cell wall the synthesis of teichoic acid is closely associated with that of peptidoglycan.

In the Gram-positive mycobacteria the peptidoglycan carries

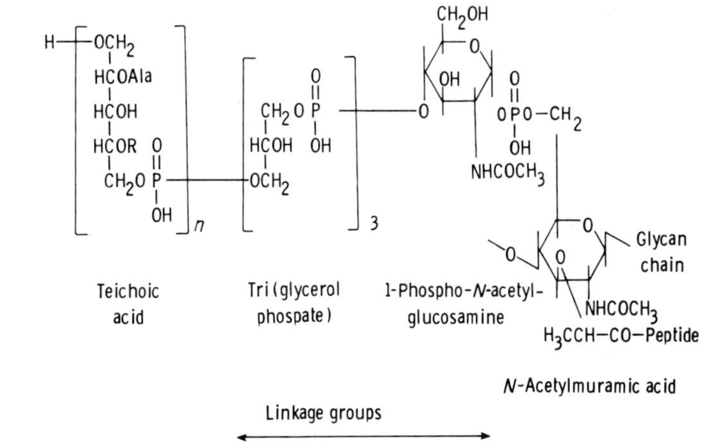

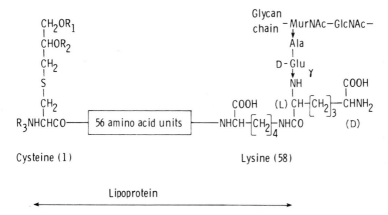

Figure 2.8 Teichoic acid and its linkage to peptidoglycan in the wall of *Staphylococcus aureus*.

quite a different polymeric attachment. Arabinogalactan is attached to the 6-position of some of the *N*-glycolylmuramic acid residues of the glycan chain through a phosphate ester group. Mycolic acids (complex, very-long-chain fatty acids) are attached by ester links to the C-5 position of arabinose residues of the arabinogalactan. The wall thus has a high lipid content.

In *E.coli* and related bacteria the peptidoglycan carries lipoprotein as a substituent (Fig. 2.9). The lipoprotein consists of a polypeptide chain of 58 amino acid units of known sequence with lysine at the

Figure 2.9 Lipoprotein and its linkage to peptidoglycan in the envelope of *Escherichia coli*.

C-terminal and cysteine at the *N*-terminal. This is attached to the 2-carboxyl group of *meso*-2,6-diaminopimelic acid in a peptide side chain of *E.coli* peptidoglycan which has lost both D-alanine groups. Attachment is by an amide link with the ε-amino group in the terminal lysine of the polypeptide. At the opposite end of the polypeptide chain the cysteine amino group carries a long-chain fatty acid joined as an amide, and its sulphur atom forms a thioether link with a long-chain diacylglycerol.

Lipoprotein occurs in enteric bacteria other than *E.coli*, but it may not be common to all Gram-negative bacteria. Small amounts have been detected with some difficulty in *Proteus mirabilis* and it could not be found in *Pseudomonas fluorescens*.

Antibiotics having a primary action on peptidoglycan biosynthesis

The conclusion that a particular antibiotic owes its antibacterial activity to interference with peptidoglycan biosynthesis rests on a number of lines of evidence:

(a) Bacteria suspended in a medium of high osmotic pressure are protected from concentrations of the antibiotic that would cause lysis and death in a normal medium. Under these conditions the cells lose the stiffening action of the peptidoglycan and assume a spherical shape; they are then known as spheroplasts. These retain an undamaged cytoplasmic membrane but their wall is deficient or considerably modified. Spheroplasts are in principle viable and if the antibiotic is removed they can sometimes divide and produce progeny having normal walls.

(b) A number of species of bacteria lack walls containing peptidoglycan. These include the mycoplasmas, the halophilic bacteria tolerant of high salt concentrations and the L-forms of bacteria where the normal wall structure is greatly modified. If a compound inhibits the growth of common bacteria but fails to affect bacteria of these special types, it probably owes its activity to interference with peptidoglycan synthesis.

(c) Sub-inhibitory concentrations of these antibiotics often cause accumulation in the culture medium of uridine nucleotides of *N*-acetylmuramic acid with varying numbers of amino acid residues attached. These compounds represent intermediates in the early stages of peptidoglycan biosynthesis. When an antibiotic causes a block at an early point in the reaction sequence it is not surprising to find accumulation of the intermediate immediately preceding the block. However, quantities of muramic acid nucleotides are also found in bacteria treated with antibiotics that are known to affect

Phosphomycin   Cycloserine

Figure 2.10 Antibiotics affecting early stages in the biosynthesis of peptidoglycan.

later stages in peptidoglycan biosynthesis. It seems that all the biosynthetic steps associated with the membrane are closely interlocked,
and inhibition of any one of them leads to accumulation of the last
water-soluble precursor, UDP-*N*-acetylmuramyl pentapeptide (V,
Fig. 2.5).

Individual antibiotics having this type of action will now be
considered.

Phosphomycin (Phosphonomycin)

This antibiotic has the remarkably simple structure shown in Fig. 2.10.
It acts on infections caused by both Gram-positive and Gram-negative
bacteria and its toxicity seems to be small. So far it has achieved only
limited use in clinical practice. Its inhibitory action is exerted on the
first step of peptidoglycan biosynthesis, namely the condensation of
UDP-*N*-acetylglucosamine (I) with phosphoenol pyruvate by means
of a transferase giving the intermediate (II) that subsequently yields
UDP-*N*-acetylmuramic acid (III) on reduction (Fig. 2.4). This is
demonstrated by tests on the isolated enzyme system. Moreover the
inhibitory action of phosphomycin towards *Enterobacter cloacae*
can be reversed by the UDP-muramyl tripeptide or pentapeptide
intermediates characteristic of that organism, indicating that the
block must be at an earlier step in the biosynthesis.

Cycloserine

This antibiotic also has a simple structure (Fig. 2.10). It is active
against a number of bacterial species but has found practical use only
in the treatment of tuberculosis. Even here, since disturbances of the
central nervous system are recognized side effects in some patients, it
is only a reserve drug, used when resistance precludes the use of
other antitubercular agents. Cycloserine shows the usual effects that
characterize compounds acting on peptidoglycan biosynthesis, and
when cultures of *S. aureus* are grown with subinhibitory concen-

trations of cycloserine considerable amounts of the murein precursor (IV) (Fig. 2.5) accumulate in the medium. This suggests a blockage in the biosynthesis immediately beyond this point. Examination of its effects on enzymes present in cell wall extracts showed cycloserine to inhibit both alanine racemase and D-alanyl-D-alanine synthetase, the two enzymes concerned in making the dipeptide for completion of the pentapeptide side chain. Molecular models demonstrated that cycloserine was structurally related to one possible conformation of D-alanine, so its inhibitory action on these enzymes appeared to be a classical example of isosteric interference.

The observation that the action of cycloserine is specifically antagonized by the addition of D-alanine to the growth medium supported the postulated site of action. Tests on the synthetase enzymes isolated from different bacterial species showed that the affinity of cycloserine for the synthetase was much greater than that of the natural substrate, the ratio of K_m to K_i being about 100.

Source of synthetase	K_m for D-alanine mM	K_i for cycloserine mM
Staphylococcus aureus	3-5	0.02-0.04
Streptococcus faecalis	0.66	0.025
Mycobacterium tuberculosis	2.0	0.03

In a compound acting purely as a competitive enzyme inhibitor, this sort of K_m/K_i ratio is probably essential for the exhibition of useful antibacterial activity. The greater affinity of cycloserine for the enzyme may be connected with its rigid structure. This could permit a particularly accurate fit to the active centre of the enzyme, either in the state existing when the enzyme is uncombined with its substrate or in some modified conformation which is assumed during the normal enzymic reaction. Rigid structures of narrow molecular specificity are common among antimicrobial agents and similar considerations may apply to other types of action; this theme will recur in later sections.

Cycloserine enters the bacterial cell by active transport (see Chapter 7). This allows the antibiotic to reach higher concentrations in the cell than in the medium and adds considerably to its antibacterial efficacy.

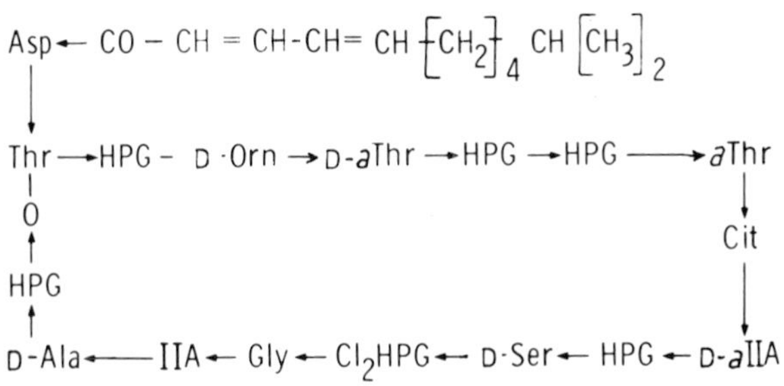

$$\text{Asp} \leftarrow CO - CH = CH - CH = CH \left[CH_2\right]_4 CH \left[CH_3\right]_2$$

$$\text{Thr} \longrightarrow \text{HPG} - \text{D} \cdot \text{Orn} \longrightarrow \text{D-aThr} \longrightarrow \text{HPG} \longrightarrow \text{HPG} \longrightarrow \text{aThr}$$

O

HPG   Cit

$$\text{D-Ala} \longleftarrow \text{IIA} \longleftarrow \text{Gly} \longleftarrow \text{Cl}_2\text{HPG} \longleftarrow \text{D-Ser} \longleftarrow \text{HPG} \longleftarrow \text{D-aIIA}$$

Figure 2.11 Enduracidin A. Abbreviations: HPG *p*-hydroxyphenylglycine; Cl$_2$HPG 3, 5-dichloro-4-hydroxyphenylglycine; Cit citrulline; Orn ornithine; IIA iminoimidazolinylaminopropionic acid:

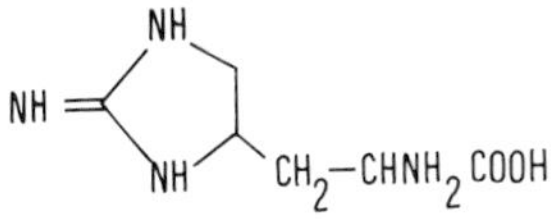

a indicates the *allo* configuration. Amino acid residues are L unless otherwise indicated.

Vancomycin, enduracidin, moenomycin and tunicamycin

The first three of these compounds are conveniently considered together because they affect that part of peptidoglycan biosynthesis which occurs while the intermediates are bound to the cytoplasmic membrane, though each probably affects different parts of this complex process. Each compound is chosen as a representative of a chemically related group of antibiotics. All are substances of relatively high molecular weight and act mainly against Gram-positive bacteria. They are effective against infections when given by injection but are not absorbed by mouth. This, and toxic side effects especially kidney damage, have limited their clinical usefulness.

Enduracidin A (Fig. 2.11) is a polypeptide antibiotic containing a number of unusual amino acid residues. It is cyclized through an ester bond and has a side chain terminated by an unsaturated acid group. Its name reflects its persistence in the animal body; a single dose maintains effective blood levels for more than 24 hours. With peptidoglycan-synthesizing systems, either complete cells or as cell-free preparations to which UDP-*N*-acetylmuramyl pentapeptide and UDP-*N*-acetylglucosamine have been added as preformed substrates, addition of enduracidin leads to accumulation of the lipid intermediate VIII (Fig. 2.6). The block in biosynthesis thus appears to occur beyond this point.

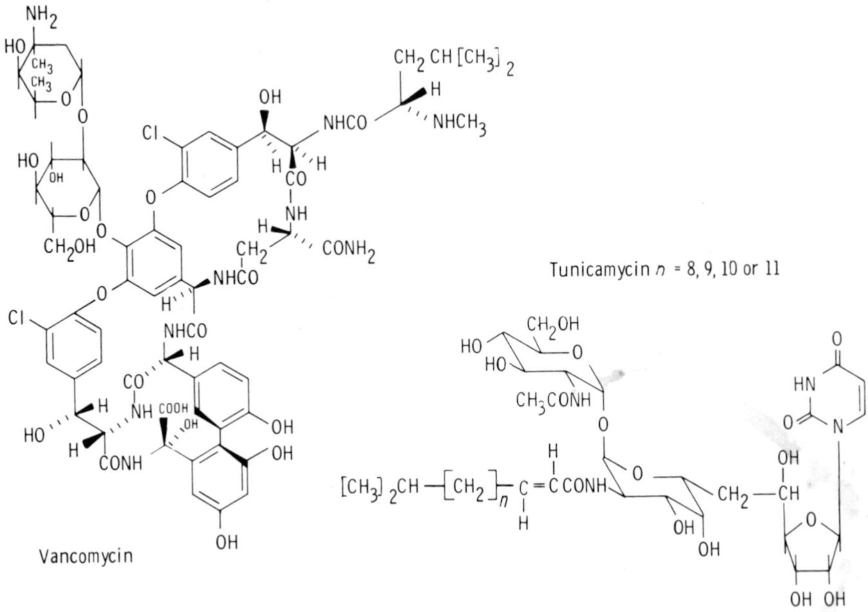

Figure 2.12 Vancomycin and tunicamycin.

Vancomycin (Fig. 2.12) has found particular use against trouble-some intestinal infections due to *Clostridium difficile*. This organism sometimes multiplies and produces toxins when the usual gut flora have been largely eliminated by the use of broad-spectrum anti-biotics. Vancomycin and the related ristocetin produce similar effects to enduracidin on peptidoglycan-synthesizing systems. The action of vancomycin depends on its ability to bind specifically to the D-alanyl-D-alanine group on the peptide side chain of one of the membrane-bound intermediates in peptidoglycan synthesis (compounds VI to IX in Fig. 2.6). Moenomycin is representative of another large group of long-acting antibiotics having molecular weights of about 1800 and possessing one phosphorus atom per molecule. Various hydrolytic products including aminohexoses have been identified, but the full structure is still unknown. One fragment is moenocinol (Fig. 2.13), a non-isoprenoid branched-chain

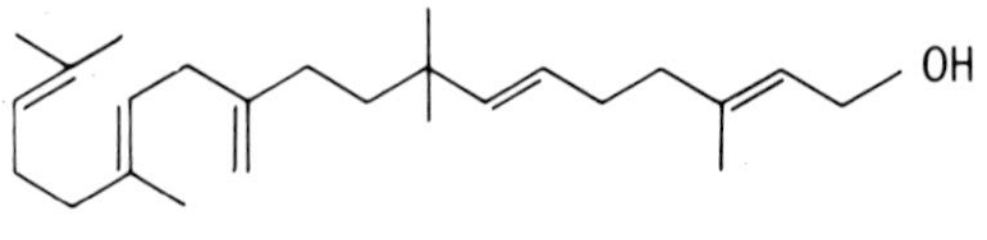

Figure 2.13 Moenocinol. A degradation product from moenomycin.

unsaturated alcohol. This structure combined with the presence of a phosphate ester group has suggested some interaction with processes involving undecaprenyl phosphate. In peptidoglycan-synthesizing systems moenomycin resembles enduracidin in causing an accumulation of lipid intermediates.

Tunicamycin (Fig. 2.12) is an antibiotic of no therapeutic value, but is widely used as a biochemical tool. It inhibits the polymerization of carbohydrates in processes involving a long-chain acyl phosphate. These reactions occur in plant and animal tissues as well as in bacteria. Tunicamycin inhibits the linkage of compound V (Fig. 2.6) to undecaprenyl phosphate, but does not prevent the next step, the conversion of VI to VII. It also inhibits the synthesis of teichoic acid.

Penicillins, cephalosporins and other β-lactam antibiotics

Penicillin was the first antibiotic to be discovered and used. It is one of a group of compounds known as the β-lactam antibiotics which are unrivalled in the treatment of bacterial infections. Their only serious defect is their characteristic of inducing immunological sensitization in a small proportion of patients, a side effect which precludes their use in those affected. The original penicillins isolated directly from mould fermentations were mixtures of compounds having different side chains. Addition of phenylacetic acid to the fermentation medium improved the yield of penicillin and ensured that the product was substantially a single compound known as penicillin G or benzyl penicillin (Fig. 2.14). The first successful variant was obtained by replacing phenylacetic acid by phenoxy-acetic acid as the added precursor. This gave phenoxymethyl penicillin or penicillin V (Fig. 2.14). The main advantage of this change was an improvement in the stability of the penicillin towards acid. The ready inactivation of penicillin G at low pH limited its usefulness when it was given by mouth, since a variable and often considerable fraction of the antibacterial activity was lost in the stomach. Penicillin V thus improved the reliability of oral dosing. These early penicillins, produced directly by fermentation, were intensely active against Gram-positive infections and gave excellent results in strepto-coccal and staphylococcal infections and in pneumonia. They were also very active against infections due to the Gram-negative gonococci and meningococci. These penicillins however were much less active against the more typical Gram-negative bacilli, and the concentrations required for inhibiting their growth were about a thousand times as high as for Gram-positive organisms.

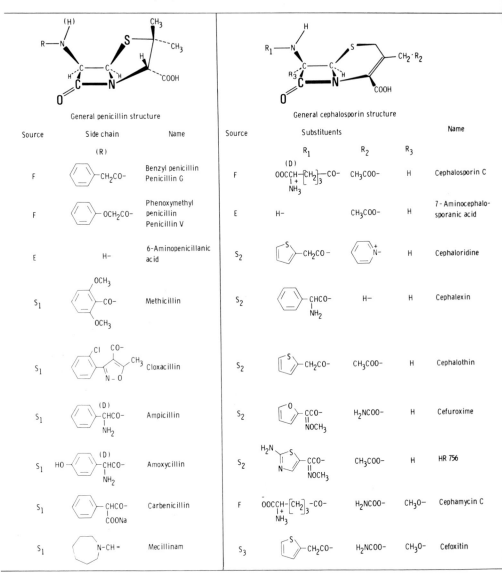

Figure 2.14 Penicillins and cephalosporins. Sources: F By fermentation: E By enzymic degradation of the corresponding fermentation product; S_1 By chemical synthesis from 6-aminopenicillanic acid; S_2 By chemical synthesis from 7-aminocephalosporanic acid; S_3 Semi-synthetically from cephamycin C.

A further advance in the versatility of the penicillins was achieved by workers of the Beecham group with the development of a method for the chemical modification of the penicillin molecule. Bacterial enzymes were found that remove the benzyl side chain from penicillin G leaving 6-aminopenicillanic acid (Fig. 2.14) which could be isolated and then acylated by chemical means. This discovery opened the way to the production of an almost unlimited number of penicillin derivatives, some of which have shown important changes of properties compared with the parent penicillin. Three types of improvement have been achieved. The value of increased stability to acids has already been mentioned, and some semi-synthetic penicillins show this property. A limitation to the use of penicillins, particularly against staphylococci, was the rapid development of resistance due to the action of the enzyme penicillinase (β-lactamase) which converts penicillin to the antibacterially inactive penicilloic acid (see Chapter 8). Some modified penicillins (e.g. methicillin and cloxacillin Fig. 2.14) are much less susceptible to attack by the commonest forms of this enzyme and are therefore useful against resistant strains. The most striking change brought about by chemical modification of the penicillin side chain is an increase of activity against Gram-negative bacteria, a property found in ampicillin, amoxycillin and carbenicillin (Fig. 2.14). The increase in this type of activity is accompanied by a lessening of activity towards Gram-positive bacteria. The compounds thus approximate more closely to the 'broad-spectrum' type of antibiotics. Ampicillin is one of the most widely used antibacterial agents. Carbenicillin finds its main use against *Pseudomonas* infections that are otherwise difficult to treat. In mecillinam (Fig. 2.14) the side chain is attached by an azomethine link rather than the usual amide bond. Here the activity spectrum of the original penicillin molecule has been completely reversed. This compound his highly active against Gram-negative bacteria but requires 50 times the concentration for an equal effect on Gram-positive organisms. It is useful in the treatment of typhoid fever.

Cephalosporin C (Fig. 2.14), isolated from a different organism from that used for penicillin production was shown to have a structure similar in its nucleus to the penicillins. The biogenesis of the nuclei in these two classes of antibiotics is now known to be identical except for the mode of closure of the sulphur-bearing ring. The penicillins have a five-membered thiazolidine ring with dimethyl substitution at position 5. In cephalosporin C the carbon atom corresponding to one of these two methyl groups forms part of the six-membered dihydrothiazine ring. Besides this similarity in structure and biogenesis, cephalosporin C and its derivatives act on peptidoglycan cross-linking in the same way as the penicillins. Cephalosporin C itself has not found substantial use as an anti-bacterial drug. It is, however, amenable to modification in a similar

stands alone, not condensed to a second ring. Sodium clavulanate, yet another structural variant, has only feeble antibiotic activity, but strongly inhibits β-lactamases. It can therefore be used in conjunction with an active β-lactam antibiotic such as ampicillin against organisms which would otherwise be resistant because of their β-lactamase activities.

Site of action of penicillins and cephalosporins

As with many other antibiotics, early attempts to discover the biochemical action of penicillin led to conflicting hypotheses. Gradually it became accepted that the primary site of action lay in the production of cell wall material, and more specifically in the biosynthesis of peptidoglycan. Even then determination of its exact point of attack proved difficult. Intensive investigation by Strominger and Tipper finally established the main features of the whole biosynthetic sequence, as already discussed, and provided evidence that penicillin acts on the transpeptidase which brings about the cross-linking (Fig. 2.7).

Evidence for this site of action rests on several different types of experiment. *S. aureus* cells were pulse-labelled with [^{14}C] glycine and peptidoglycan was isolated from their walls after growth for a further 20 minutes in unlabelled medium. The labelled glycine entered the pentaglycyl 'extending group'. The polysaccharide backbone of the peptidoglycan was broken down by an *N*-acetyl-muramidase leaving the individual muramyl peptide units linked together only by their pentaglycyl peptide chains. The product was separated on columns of Sephadex G-50 and G-25. Radioactivity was distributed in a series of peaks of increasing molecular weight representing the distribution of the pulse of [^{14}C] glycine among peptide-linked oligomers of varying size. A parallel experiment done in the presence of penicillin showed the radioactivity to be associated very largely with a single low-molecular-weight peak, presumably the uncross-linked muramyl peptide unit, with much less activity in the oligomers. The penicillin had thus inhibited the peptide cross-linking.

In another experiment 'nucleotide pentapeptide' was prepared with ^{14}C-labelled D-alanine. This was used as a substrate for a particulate enzyme preparation from *E.coli* in the presence of UDP-*N*-acetylglucosamine. This system carried out the whole biosynthesis of peptidoglycan including the final cross-linking. Peptidoglycan was obtained as an insoluble product containing ^{14}C from the penultimate D-alanine of the substrate; the terminal D-[^{14}C] alanine was released into the medium, partly from the transpeptidase cross-linking reaction and partly from a carboxypeptidase that removed terminal D-alanine

residues from cross-linked products. In a parallel experiment pencillin
was added at a concentration that would inhibit growth of *E.coli*.
Biosynthesis of peptidoglycan then proceeded only to the stage of
the linear polymer (IX Fig. 2.6) which was isolated as a high-
molecular-weight water-soluble product labelled with ^{14}C. No D-[^{14}C]
alanine was liberated because the penicillin had suppressed both the
cross-linking transpeptidase reaction and the action of DD-carboxypeptidase.

Electron micrographs of thin sections of penicillin-treated *Bacillus
megaterium* show abnormalities consistent with the accumulation of
linear polymer in place of the normal cross-linked peptidoglycan.
This is seen particularly during the formation of the septum which
precedes the division of a cell. In Fig. 2.16 the appearance of a cross-

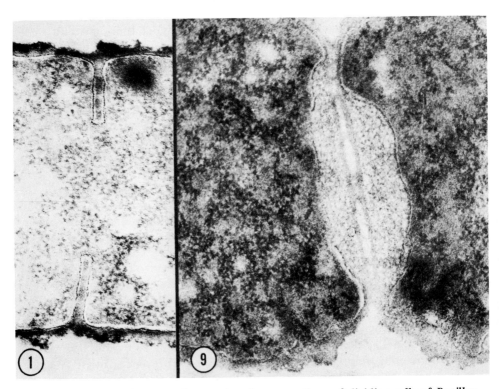

Figure 2.16 Electron micrographs of cross-sections of dividing cells of *Bacillus
megaterium*. Picture (1) shows the septum forming in a normal cell. Picture (9)
shows cell division after treatment with penicillin. Note the accumulation of
fibrous material at the growing point. Reprinted by permission of The Rockefeller
University Press from P. FITZJAMES and R. HANCOCK (1965), *J. Cell Biol.*,
26 657.

section of normal septum formation is contrasted with a cross-section from a penicillin-treated cell. The normal wall is replaced by masses of fibrous material.

Release of uncross-linked peptidoglycan into the medium has been observed after penicillin treatment of growing cultures of *Micrococcus luteus* and a mutant of *Bacillus licheniformis*.

Despite intensive research, the transpeptidase which is the basis of penicillin attack has defied isolation. Its activity can be demonstrated in crude particulate wall-membrane preparations, but all attempts to purify it have led to inactivation. This may be due to inhibition by the detergents used to separate the protein from the membrane, or may be due to a requirement for particular spatial relationships between enzyme and substrate which exist on the membrane but are lost in solution. Even so, examination of related enzymes throws much light on the probable structure and properties of the elusive membrane transpeptidase. The enzymes widely studied have been two extracellular DD-carboxypeptidases produced by *Streptomyces* species and carboxypeptidases solubilized from the membrane of *E.coli* or *B.stearothermophilus*. The streptomyces enzymes display some transpeptidase activity besides their high carboxypeptidase activity. The relationship between these two enzymic actions has been shown with model substrates. The transpeptidase reaction

$$Ac_2 \text{ L-Lys} \cdot \text{D-Ala} \cdot \text{D-Ala} + \text{Gly} \cdot \text{Gly} \xrightarrow[\text{reaction}]{\text{Transpeptidase}} Ac_2 \text{ L-Lys} \cdot \text{D-Ala} \cdot \text{Gly} \cdot \text{Gly}$$

Donor

$$+ \text{ D-Ala}$$

$$\searrow + \text{ H}_2\text{O} \xrightarrow[\text{reaction}]{\text{Carboxypeptidase}} Ac_2 \text{ L-Lys} \cdot \text{D-Ala}$$

Acceptors

$$+ \text{ D-Ala}$$

$(Ac_2 \text{ L-Lys} = NN'\text{-diacetyl-L-lysine})$

which is exactly analogous to cross-linking of peptidoglycan (Fig. 2.7) is competitive with the carboxypeptidase reaction and is favoured by high concentrations of the substrates. Carboxypeptidases have been used to show the nature of interaction of a penicillin or cephalosporin (I) with the enzyme (E). This may be represented as:

$$E + I \underset{k_2}{\overset{k_1}{\rightleftharpoons}} EI \xrightarrow{k_3} EI^* \xrightarrow{k_4} E + \begin{array}{l}\text{degraded}\\\text{inhibitor}\end{array}$$

The first reaction is reversible binding to the enzyme. The second stage, involving chemical modification of the inhibitor with covalent binding to the enzyme, is irreversible as is the final stage of enzyme release. For high antibacterial activity k_3 should be rapid, preventing release of I through reversal of the initial binding, and k_4 should be slow to maintain the enzyme in the inactive EI* form and to avoid significant reactivation. Measurements show that the widely used β-lactam antibiotics show just such characteristics, and this scheme goes far to explain their outstanding effectiveness. There is every reason to suppose that the inactivation mechanism is the same with cross-linking transpeptidases as with DD-carboxypeptidases. The nature of the end products of penicillin degradation depends on the enzyme involved. It may be a simple opening of the β-lactam ring to give the penicilloate (Fig. 8.5) or there may be more extensive breakdown leading to the production, from benzyl penicillin, of phenylacetylglycine. Those enzymes which yield penicilloate are equivalent to slow-acting β-lactamases. Quite possibly active β-lactamases are relatives of carboxypeptidases and transpeptidases in which reaction k_4 is rapid instead of very slow.

It seemed likely that the mechanism of action of DD-carboxypeptidases and cross-linking transpeptidases resembled that of certain esterases and amidases. These enzymes possess specially reactive groups, associated with their active centres, which undergo transient acylation in the course of enzymic action. Antibiotics containing a β-lactam ring behave chemically as acylating agents, reacting to produce penicilloyl derivatives. The action of penicillin on these enzymes might thus involve acylation of the enzymically active site with formation of the rather stable inactive complex EI*. This explanation has received strong support from experiments with purified DD-carboxypeptidases from *Bacillus stearothermophilus* and *Bacillus subtilis*. The enzyme was allowed to react briefly with $[^{14}C]$ benzyl penicillin or with a substrate analogue $[^{14}C]$ Ac$_2$ L-Lys· D-Ala-D-actate; D-lactic acid is the exact hydroxyl analogue of D-alanine, and use of this derivative enables the transient enzyme reaction intermediate to be trapped. The treated enzyme was then broken down into peptide units either by cyanogen bromide or pepsin. In products from the *B.stearothermophilus* enzyme, radioactivity was found in a peptide with 40 amino acid residues. This was sequenced, and the label was shown to be associated with the same specific serine residue, whether the reactant was benzyl penicillin or the substrate analogue. Similar results were found with the *B.subtilis* enzyme from which a labelled 14 unit peptide was isolated. This peptide showed strong homology with 14 residues of the *B.stearothermophilus* peptide and the label was associated with the corresponding serine residue. Thus for these enzymes penicillin apparently binds to the active site and acylates the same serine as the substrate. Unlike the substrate, the degraded penicillin is only released very slowly (reaction k_4 in the scheme above) and thus blocks further access of substrate to the site. Again the extension of this result to the effect of penicillin on cross-linking transpeptidase seems reasonable but remains to be proved.

How can this action of penicillin be related to its structure? The most widely quoted explanation is due to Strominger. It depends on the similarity of the spatial orientation of the principal atoms and polar groups in the penicillin nucleus to one particular orientation of the D-alanyl-D-alanine end group of the pentapeptide side chain of peptidoglycan precursors (see Fig. 2.17). When the two structures are compared, the peptide bond between the alanine units is seen to correspond in position to the lactam group in the four-membered

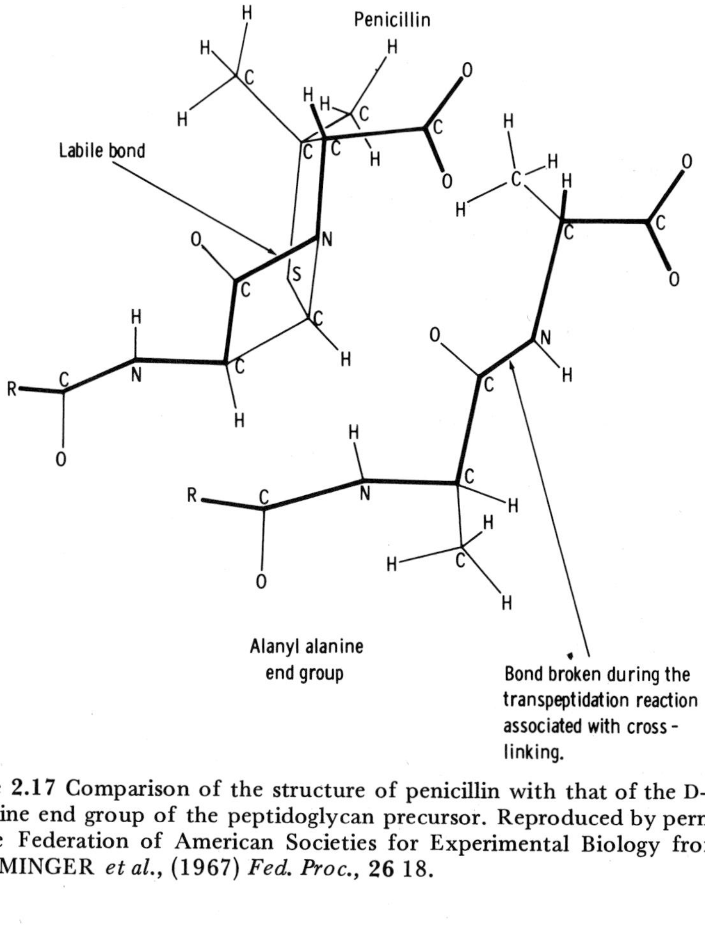

Figure 2.17 Comparison of the structure of penicillin with that of the D-alanyl-D-alanine end group of the peptidoglycan precursor. Reproduced by permission of the Federation of American Societies for Experimental Biology from J.L. STROMINGER *et al.*, (1967) *Fed. Proc.*, 26 18.

ring of penicillin responsible for its acylating properties. Such a group bound to the cross-linking transpeptidase close to its active centre could well usurp the acylating function implicit in the normal reaction of the substrate with the enzyme. When the structures (illustrated in Fig. 2.17) are compared more critically it becomes apparent that the agreement between them is imperfect, but can be much improved if the peptide bond of the D-alanyl-D-alanine end group is represented not in its normal planar form but twisted nearly 45° out of plane. This may imply that the conformation of the penicillin molecule resembles the transition state of the substrate rather than its resting form. During the enzymic transpeptidation the peptide bond quite possibly undergoes this sort of distortion. A further discrepancy is that the usual penicillins lack a methyl group in a position corresponding to that of the penultimate D-alanine residue. A penicillin with a methyl group in the appropriate 6-position, which would be expected to give a better fit, was made and shown to be antibacterially inactive, though oddly the 6-methoxy derivatives show good activity. Clearly there is still much to be learnt about the exact relationship between structure and mode of action. The rigidity of the bicyclic ring structures of the penicillins and cephalosporins maintains the principal binding groups in fixed relative conformation. This may be an important feature in binding to the active site.

Actions of β-lactam antibacterials on gram-negative bacteria

The action of β-lactam antibiotics on Gram-positive cocci appears to be straightforward inhibition of the cross-linking transpeptidase. With Gram-negative enteric bacteria the matter is more complex. Progress has been made in understanding the action of β-lactam antibiotics on *E.coli* by binding studies. Preparations from *E.coli* membranes show the presence of six proteins capable of binding penicillin. These proteins vary in molecular weight, enzymic activity and apparent function. Their properties are summarized in Table 2.1.

Only proteins 4, 5 and 6 have been purified in an enzymically active form. The possible function of these carboxypeptidases in limiting the cross-linking of Gram-negative peptidoglycan and in the attachment of lipoprotein has already been discussed. Different β-lactam antibiotics vary in the relative strengths of their binding to proteins 1, 2 and 3. There are corresponding differences in their effects on cell morphology as revealed by electron microscopy (Fig. 2.18). Protein 1 is regarded as the main cross-linking trans-peptidase, and compounds which bind most strongly to this cause

Table 2.1 Penicillin-binding proteins from *E.coli*

Protein No.	10^{-3} x Mol. wt.	Proposed enzymic activity	Proposed function
1	91	Transpeptidase (wall)	Cell elongation
2	66	?	Cell-shape maintenance
3	60	Transpeptidase (septum)	Septum formation
4	49	Carboxypeptidase II	Attachment of lipoprotein
5	42	DD-Carboxypeptidase }	Control of cross-linking
6	40	,, ,,	

lysis of the cells at the lowest antibacterial concentration. Compounds such as cephalexin, which bind more strongly to protein 3, inhibit the formation of septa and lead to the formation of filaments, which are greatly elongated cells (Fig. 2.18c). This distinction in the action of β-lactams associated with differences in binding behaviour adds further weight to the supposition, discussed above, that different mechanisms may be involved in synthesis of peptidoglycan for cell extension compared with its synthesis for septum formation. Yet another variation is found with mecillinam which binds almost exclusively to protein 2, and causes cells to assume an abnormal ovoid shape (Fig. 2.18b). This compound is also unusual in other ways. It does not inhibit cross-linking in membrane preparations and, unlike other β-lactam antibiotics, it fails to inhibit DD-carboxy-peptidase. In spite of this it has high antibacterial activity against *E.coli*. A mixture of cephalexin and mecillinam produces filamentous cells with bulges (Fig. 2.18d), and a similar effect is seen with compounds, e.g. ampicillin, which bind about equally to proteins 2 and 3. Evidently β-lactams can affect more than one process in *E.coli*, though some of these are poorly understood. Probably in normal use a combined effect on several systems is involved.

Bacitracin

Bacitracin, a polypeptide antibiotic (Fig. 2.19), is too toxic for systemic treatment but is sometimes used locally to kill Gram-positive bacteria, e.g. in surgery of the colon. Its effect on peptidoglycan biosynthesis depends upon its ability to bind specifically to polyprenyl pyrophosphates in the presence of magnesium ions. In the formation of the linear peptidoglycan (IX, Fig. 2.6) the membrane-bound undecaprenyl pyrophosphate is released. Normally this is converted by a pyrophosphatase to the corresponding phosphate which thus becomes available for reaction

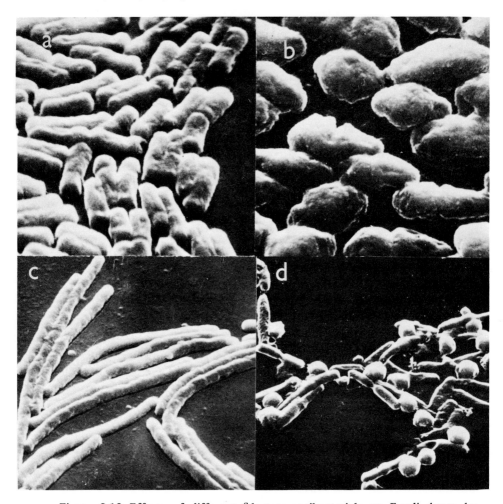

Figure 2.18 Effects of different β-lactam antibacterials on *E.coli* shown by scanning electron microscopy. **a**, Normal culture. Other pictures show cells after 60 min treatment with the compounds indicated. **b**, Mecillinam (10 μg/ml). **c** Cephalexin (32 μg/ml). **d** Mecillinam (10 μg/ml) and cephalexin (32 μg/ml). Magnifications: a 11 000; b 12 000; c 5 800; d 4 00. Reprinted by permission of the University of Chicago Press and the authors, D. GREENWOOD and F. O'GRADY (1973), from *J. Infect. Dis.*, **128** 793.

with another molecule of UDPMurNAc pentapeptide (V). Complex formation of the pyrophosphate with bacitracin blocks this process and so eventually halts the synthesis of peptidoglycan. Bacitracin also inhibits sterol biosynthesis in animal tissues through complex formation with intermediates such as farnesyl pyrophosphate.

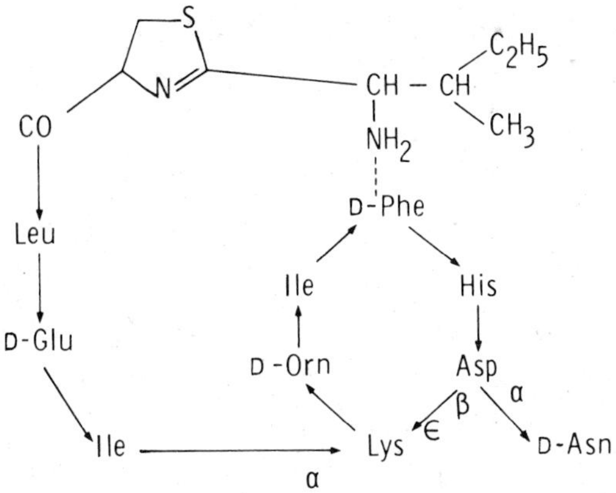

Figure 2.19 Bacitracin A.

Other antibiotics affecting wall synthesis

Cerulenin

This compound (Fig. 2.20) is active against a range of bacteria, yeasts and fungi. Although not unduly toxic to animals, it has not been developed as an agent against microbial infections, but its unusual mode of action makes it a useful biochemical tool. It inhibits the synthesis of long-chain fatty acids by blocking β-ketoacyl acyl carrier protein synthetase. The effect is readily demonstrated by inhibition

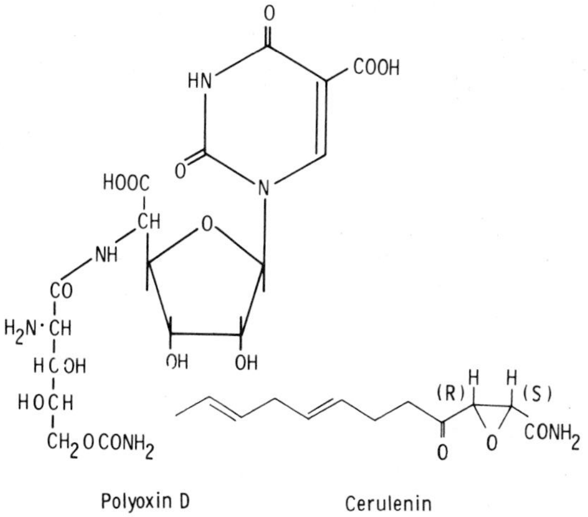

Polyoxin D   Cerulenin

Figure 2.20 Polyoxin D and cerulenin.

of incorporation of labelled acetate into all cell components containing fatty acids. This affects many organisms by stopping the synthesis
of membrane phospholipids. In Gram-negative bacteria the outer
membrane is also affected by the failure to form lipopolysaccharide
and lipoprotein. The action of cerulenin is purely bacteriostatic;
inhibited cells washed free of the compound resume fatty acid
production and grow normally. The inhibitory effect of cerulenin
can be partly countered by providing cells with an exogenous source
of long-chain fatty acids.

Polyoxins — inhibitors of fungal wall synthesis

The walls of fungi do not contain peptidoglycan, so antibiotics which
rely for their effect on inhibition of synthesis of this cell component
are inactive against fungi. In fungal walls the rigid structural feature
is a poly(N-acetylglucosamine) known as chitin. A family of antibiotics, the polyoxins (Fig. 2.20), that are specifically active against
fungi cause swelling of their cell walls and can be used to produce
fungal protoplasts. They act as powerful competitive inhibitors of
the synthesis of chitin from N-acetylglucosamine; for an isolated
chitin synthetase from *Mucor rouxii* the K_m for UDP-N-acetylglucosamine was 0.5 mM whilst K_i for polyoxin D was 0.6 μM.
Treatment of *Alternaria kikuchiana* with polyoxin caused an
inhibition of the incorporation of labelled glucosamine into chitin
and an abnormal accumulation of UDP-N-acetylglucosamine in the
cells. The polyoxins are much more active against filamentous fungi,
which are particularly dependent on chitin production, than against
the yeast forms.

Further reading

The cell wall and its constitutents

H. NIKAIDO and T. NAKAE (1979), 'The outer membrane of Gram-negative
bacteria', in *Adv. Microb. Physiol.*, **20**, 163.
J.M. di RIENZO, K. NAKAMURA and M. INOUYE (1978), 'Outer membrane
proteins of Gram-negative bacteria', in *Annu. Rev. Biochem.*, **47**, 481.
J. COLEY, E. TARELLI, A.R. ARCHIBALD and J. BADDILEY (1978), 'The
linkage between teichoic acid and peptidoglycan in bacterial cell walls', in
FEBS Lett., **88**, 1.

Biogenesis of the cell wall

D.J. TIPPER and A. WRIGHT (1979), 'The structure and biosynthesis of cell
walls', in *The Bacteria*, **8**, 291.

H.J. ROGERS (1979), 'Biogenesis of the wall in bacterial morphogenesis', in *Adv. Microb. Physiol.*, **19**, 1.
D. MIRELMAN, Y. YASHOUV-GAN and U. SCHWARTZ (1976), 'Peptidoglycan biosynthesis in a thermosensitive division mutant of *Escherichia coli*', in *Biochemistry*, **15**, 1781.

β-Lactam antibiotics

Compounds and use
E.H. FLYNN (ed), *Cephalosporins and Penicillins. Chemistry and Biology* (Academic Press, 1972).
J.H.C. NAYLER (1973), 'Advances in penicillin research', in *Adv. Drug Res.*, **7**, 1.
D.R. OWENS, D.K. LUSCOMBE, A.D. RUSSELL and P.J. NICHOLS (1975), 'The cephalosporin group of antibiotics', in *Adv. Pharmacol. Chemother.*, **13**, 83.
L.D. CAMA and B.G. CHRISTENSEN (1978), 'Structure-activity relationships of "non-classical" β-lactam antibiotics', in *Annu. Rep. Med. Chem.*, **13**, 149.
L.P. GARROD (1974), 'Choice among penicillins and cephalosporins', in *Brt. Med. J.*, 1974 (iii), 96.
G.T. STEWART (1973), 'Allergy to penicillin and related antibiotics: antigenic and immunochemical mechanism', in *Annu. Rev. Pharmacol.*, **13**, 309.

Biochemical action
P.M. BLUMBERG and J.L. STROMINGER (1974), 'Interaction of penicillin with the bacterial cell: penicillin-binding proteins and penicillin-sensitive enzymes', in *Annu. Rev. Biochem.*, **38**, 291.
J. - M. GHUYSEN (1979), 'The concept of the penicillin target from 1965 until today', in *J. Gen. Microbiol.*, **101**, 13.
J. - M. GHUYSEN (1979), 'Use of model enzymes in determining the mode of action of penicillins and Δ^3-cephalosporins', in *Annu. Rev. Biochem.*, **48**, 73.

Other antibiotics affecting wall synthesis

M.R.J. SALTON and A. TOMASZ (eds), 'Mode of action of antibiotics on microbial walls and membranes', in *Ann. N.Y. Acad. Sci.*, **235**, 1974.
A. GALLEGO and J.M. RUBIO (eds), 'Fosfomycin' (a symposium on phosphomycin), in *Chemotherapy* 23, *Supp. 1*, 1.
S. ŌMURA (1976), 'The antibiotic cerulenin, a novel tool for biochemistry as an inhibitor of fatty acid synthesis', in *Bacteriol. Rev.*, **40**, 681.
V. FARKAŠ (1979), 'Biosynthesis of cell walls of fungi', in *Microbiol. Rev.*, **43**, 117.

3 Antiseptics, antibiotics and the cell membrane

Bacteria killers: antiseptics and disinfectants

The major interest throughout this book lies in antibacterial substances that can be used against bacterial infections. For this purpose the compound must normally be absorbed and must circulate in the blood. However, there is a widespread requirement in medicine and in industry for substances that kill bacteria and other micro-organisms on the surface of the body or in other places. Such products are known as disinfectants, sterilants, antiseptics or biocides, the choice of term depending on the circumstances in which they are used. 'Disinfectant' describes products intended for use in the presence of dirt and dense bacterial populations, for example in the cleaning of animal quarters or drains. 'Biocide' is used more particularly for preservatives that prevent bacterial and fungal attack on wood, paper, textiles and all kinds of organic material. 'Antiseptic' is a term usually reserved for a substance that can be safely applied to the skin with the aim of reducing the chances of infection by killing the surface bacteria. 'Sterilants' are substances used to sterilize an enclosed space; since penetration is paramount in this application sterilants are usually gaseous. However, all these terms are to some extent overlapping and interchangeable.

The requirements for a compound having disinfectant or antiseptic action differ markedly from those needed in a systemic antibacterial. Many compounds successfully used against bacterial infections do not actually kill bacteria, but only prevent their multiplication; most are inactive against non-growing bacteria. A cessation of bacterial growth is usually all that is needed in treating an infection, since the body has antibody and phagocytic defences that can soon be mobilized to remove bacteria present in relatively small numbers. Furthermore, systemic antibacterials are often active against a fairly limited range of bacteria. This is acceptable since the compound can be selected according to the nature of the infection that is being treated.

A distinction is often made between bacteriostatic and bactericidal compounds, but the division is by no means clear cut. There is no certain way of determining whether a bacterium is dead. The usual method of assessing the killing effect of an antiseptic is by measuring the 'viable count' of a treated bacterial suspension. The antiseptic is first inactivated and dilutions of the suspension are added to a rich medium. Bacteria are deemed to be alive if they give rise to colonies. However, since the formation of a visible colony requires multiplication for at least 20 generations, failure to produce a colony is rather indirect evidence of death. Many compounds are bacteriostatic at low concentrations and bactericidal at higher concentrations, and the effect may also depend on the conditions of culture. However, for antiseptics and disinfectants a bactericidal effect is required under all normal conditions of application. Such compounds must be able to kill bacteria whether they are growing or resting and must be able to deal with most of the common bacteria likely to be found in the environment.

Many of the older disinfectants are compounds of considerable chemical reactivity. Their antibacterial action presumably depends on their ability to react chemically with various groups on or in the bacterium, thus killing it. Such compounds include hydrogen peroxide, the halogens and the hypochlorites, the gaseous sterilants ethylene oxide, ozone etc. Salts and other derivatives of the heavy metals, particularly of mercury, probably owe their antibacterial effect to reaction with vital thiol groups. Although some of these substances still have important uses in disinfection, their high reactivity and toxicity limit their scope and they are not nowadays generally acceptable for the more delicate uses as antiseptics. For this purpose two main groups of compounds are used almost exclusively: the phenols and the cationic antiseptics. Although there are differences between the actions of these two classes of compound they show many common features. The literature on the mode of action of antiseptics is confused, and much of the earlier work needs revising in the light of more modern techniques. A review of the most reliable evidence suggests the following generalizations:

(1) Antiseptics bind readily to bacteria, the amount adsorbed increasing with an increasing concentration in solution. The adsorption isotherm sometimes shows a point of inflection which corresponds to the minimum bactericidal concentration: higher concentrations lead to a much greater adsorption of the compound. The most important site of adsorption is the cytoplasmic membrane. Spheroplasts or protoplasts lacking the outer cell wall layers will bind the antiseptic and may be lysed or damaged. Adsorption by isolated

cell membranes can also be demonstrated.

(2) The extent of killing of the bacteria is governed by three principal factors: (a) Concentration of the antiseptic, (b) Bacterial cell density, (c) Time of contact. The adsorption of a given amount of the compound per cell leads to the killing of a definite fraction of the bacterial population in a chosen time interval.

(3) The lowest concentration of the antiseptic that causes death of the bacteria also brings about leakage of cytoplasmic constitutents of low molecular weight. The most immediate effect is loss of potassium ions. Leakage of nucleotides is often detected by the appearance in the medium of material having an optical absorption maximum at 260 nm. Gram-positive cells show leakage of amino acids. Some loss of cytoplasmic solutes is not in itself lethal. Compounds are known that cause this effect but do not kill bacteria; moreover bacteria that have been rendered leaky by low concentrations of an antiseptic will often grow normally if they are immediately washed and placed in a nutrient medium. The increased permeability is a sign of changes in the membrane which are initially reversible but become irreversible on prolonged treatment.

(4) The necessary characteristic of antiseptics is their bactericidal action, but there is often a low and rather narrow concentration range in which their effect is bacteriostatic. At these low concentrations certain biochemical functions associated with the bacterial membrane may be inhibited.

(5) In the presence of higher concentrations of antiseptic and after prolonged treatment, the compound usually penetrates the cell and brings about extensive ill-defined damage to the biochemical mechanism.

The primary effect of these antiseptics on the cytoplasmic membrane is thus established beyond doubt, but secondary actions on cytoplasmic processes are less defined and may vary from one compound to another. Examples of evidence of action for particular compounds will be given as illustrations.

Phenols

Crude mixtures of cresols solubilized by soap or alkali and originally introduced as 'lysol' are still used as rough disinfectants. They need to be applied at high concentrations and are irritant and toxic. For more refined applications as antiseptics chlorinated cresols or xylenols are commonly used, as in the well-known household antiseptic 'Dettol'. These compounds are less active than the cationic antiseptics against staphylococci and pseudomonads. Hexachlorophene (Fig 3.1)

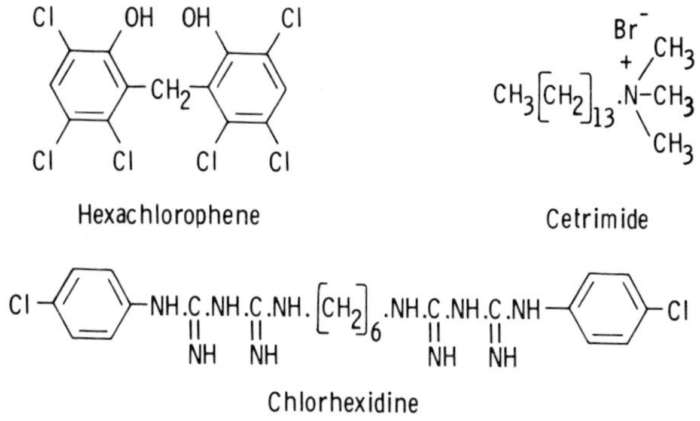

Figure 3.1 Synthetic antiseptics. The formula for cetrimide shows the main component in the preparations normally sold. Homologues with other chain lengths, especially C_{16}, are also present.

is a different kind of phenolic antiseptic. It acts only slowly, but binds strongly to the skin. It was used widely in surgical soaps and antiperspirant preparations. However, absorption through the skin can cause damage to the central nervous system, particularly in infants, and use of the compound is now severely restricted.

Hexachlorophene at bactericidal concentrations causes release of cytoplasmic components absorbing at 260 nm. A change in permeability to compounds external to the cell can be demonstrated using *N*-tolyl-l-naphthylamine-8-sulphonic acid (tolylperi acid), a compound that fluoresces strongly when it binds to proteins. This compound does not penetrate into normal bacteria, but bacteria treated with hexachlorophene absorb it and show a brilliant fluorescence. The uptake of 3,5,3′, 4′-tetrachlorosalicylanilide by *Bacilius megaterium* has been studied with the aid of ^{14}C-labelled material. Cell membranes were isolated and freed from other cellular components; they were shown to carry the whole of the radioactivity bound by the cells. The same compound tested at sub-lethal concentrations on *Staphylococcus aureus* caused a marked inhibition of oxygen consumption. This was interpreted as evidence of a direct effect on the respiratory mechanism which is associated with the membrane. Inhibition of other biochemical functions, e.g. fermentation, required higher concentrations which caused cytoplasmic leakage and cell death.

Cationic antiseptics

This classification covers a number of compounds differing considerably in chemical type. Their common features are the presence of strongly basic groups attached to a fairly massive lipophilic molecule. Although antiseptic action is found quite widely in compounds having these characteristics the degree of activity is sharply dependent on structure within any particular group. For instance in cetrimide (Fig. 3.1) the length of the main alkyl chain is 14 carbon atoms and the activity of other compounds in the same series falls off markedly with longer or shorter chains. Cetrimide combines excellent detergent properties with a useful antiseptic action, although it is not very potent against *Proteus* and *Pseudomonas* species. Experiments with *Escherichia coli* labelled with ^{32}P have shown that with increasing concentrations of cetrimide loss of cell viability closely parallels the degree of leakage of radioactivity from the bacteria. An effect on bacterial growth however is noticeable at concentrations that affect neither viability nor permeability.

One of the best and most widely used of the cationic antiseptics is chlorhexidine (Fig. 3.1). This compound has two strongly basic groups, both biguanides; it is often formulated as the digluconate which has good solubility in water. Chlorhexidine is much less surface active than cetrimide and has little detergent action. However, it acts against a wide range of bacteria at concentrations between 10 and 50 μg/ml. Its toxicity is low and it has so little irritancy that it can be used on the most sensitive mucosal surfaces. During recent years it has found an application in oral hygiene. Periodic rinsing of the mouth with chlorhexidine solution greatly reduces the population of *Streptococcus mutans* on the teeth. This minimizes the production of dental plaque and reduces periodontal infections that give rise to gingivitis. It also decreases the incidence of some types of caries. An important feature of this action is the strong binding of chlorhexidine to the tissues in the mouth with subsequent slow release which maintains an antibacterial action over an extended period. The compound also binds to the teeth and if used too freely will cause the deposition of unsightly though removable stain. Preliminary reports suggest that chlorhexidine, used in an eye lotion, may provide a cheap and effective way of controlling trachoma. This disease, due to infection by *Chlamydia trachomatis*, causes widespread blindness in Africa.

Chlorhexidine shows effects on the cytoplasmic membrane characteristic of cationic antiseptics. At concentrations that just prevent growth of *Streptoccocus faecalis* it inhibits the adenosine triphosphatase of the membrane. The effect can be shown on isolated membrane or on the solubilized enzyme derived from it. A similar concentration of chlorhexidine inhibits the net uptake of potassium ions by the intact cells, and the two effects are thought to be inter-

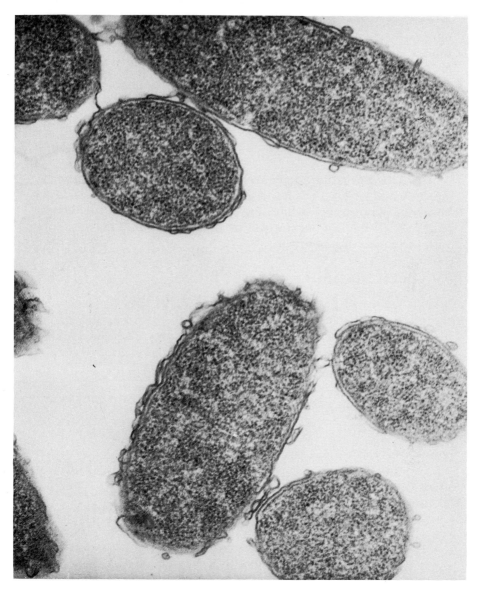

Figure 3.2 Electron micrograph of a cross-section of an *E.coli* cell after treatment with a low concentration (30 μg/ml) of chlorhexidine, showing 'blistering' of the cell wall. We thank Mr A. Davies and Mrs M. Bentley for this picture.

dependent. When bacteria are treated with a range of concentrations of chlorhexidine and then examined for leakage of cytoplasmic solutes, the degree of leakage increases with concentration up to a maximum and then declines at higher concentrations. Electron microscopy shows that the cells from these higher levels of chlorhexidine treatment are grossly altered. The increased membrane permeability apparently allows the antiseptic to enter the cytoplasm and to cause precipitation of the nucleic acid and proteins. Under these circumstances leakage is probably prevented by simple mechanical blockage.

With Gram-negative bacteria chlorhexidine may affect the outer membrane as well as the cytoplasmic membrane.This shows itself in a 'blistering' appearance which can be seen in electron micrographs (Fig. 3.2). This phenomenon will be discussed further in connection with the action of polymyxin.

Polypeptide antibiotics

Several classes of polypeptide antibiotics are known. In two groups the effects on bacteria conform exactly with the properties already discussed for the phenolic and cationic antiseptics. They are therefore regarded as owing their primary antibacterial action to their binding

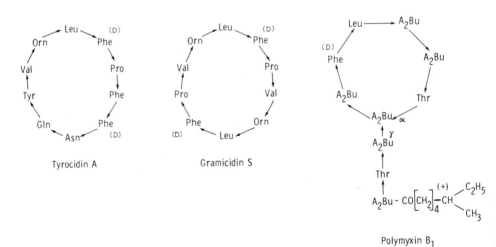

Figure 3.3 Antibiotics that produce effects on bacterial cell membranes. The usual abbreviations are used for the common amino acids. A_2Bu = 2, 4-diaminobutyric acid. Arrows show direction of the peptide bond -CO-NH-. Except where shown, all peptide linkages involve α-amino and α-carboxyl groups. Configurations are L unless otherwise indicated.

to the cytoplasmic membrane, with subsequent disturbance of its function. Both types are cyclic polypeptides. One group includes the tyrocidins and gramicidin S which are cyclic decapeptides (Fig. 3.3). These contain one or sometimes two free amino groups. They are more active against Gram-positive than against Gram-negative bacteria. The polymyxins which form the second group have a smaller polypeptide ring attached to a polypeptide chain terminating with a branched 8 or 9 carbon fatty acid residue. They have five free amino groups associated with the diaminobutyric acid units. The octapeptins have a similiar ring structure but differ in the composition of the side chain. The antibacterial action of polymyxins and octa-peptins is directed particularly against Gram-negative organisms. The cause of this selectivity is not understood. It can be dramatically altered by chemical modification. The penta-*N*-benzyl derivative is highly active against Gram-positive bacteria as shown below.

	Minimum inhibitory concentration µg/ml	
	S. aureus	E.coli
Polymyxin	120	0.3
Penta-N-*benzylpolymyxin*	1.3	5

These polypeptide antibiotics have only a minor place in medicine. The polymyxins may be used systemically in severe *Pseudomonas* infections, though there is considerable risk of kidney damage.

Polymyxin is bactericidal and acts on non-growing as well as on growing cells. At low concentrations its bactericidal action parallels the degree of release of cytoplasmic solutes. It is strongly and rapidly bound to bacteria. With *Salmonella typhimurium* the binding of 2×10^5 molecules of polymyxin per cell was shown to be bactericidal. The site of this binding has been studied with the aid of a derivative in which a fluorescent adduct is attached to one of the free amino groups (up to two of these groups may be acylated without loss of antibacterial effect). When *Bacillus megaterium*, an organism sensitive to the antibiotic, is treated with this fluorescent derivative the cells become fluorescent. Fractionation of the cells shows the fluorescence to reside almost entirely in the cytoplasmic membrane. An increase in the permeability of polymyxin-treated *Pseudomonas aeruginosa* towards solutes in the medium has been shown in an experiment with tolylperi acid similar to that described for hexachlorophene (see above). With this same organism low concentrations of polymyxin inhibit respiration, an effect also observed with some phenolic antiseptics.

Physical measurements of various kinds all tend to the conclusion that the antibacterial action of polymyxin is caused primarily by its binding to the cytoplasmic membrane. The positively charged peptide ring is thought to bind electrostatically with the anionic phosphate head groups of the membrane phospholipid, displacing magnesium ions which normally contribute to membrane stability. At the same time the fatty side chain is inserted into the hydrophobic inner region of the membrane. The effect is to disturb the normal organization of the membrane and to alter its permeability characteristics.

In Gram-negative bacteria there is a further binding to the outer membrane affecting mainly the lipopolysaccharide but with similar disorganizing effects. The gross effects of polymyxin on the outer membrane are sometimes revealed in electron micrographs as blisters similar to those caused by chlorhexidine (Fig. 3.2). The swellings may be due to an increase in the surface area of the outer leaf of the outer membrane. The parallels between the action of polymyxin and chlorhexidine are quite striking. In both, the binding and antibacterial effects can be antagonized by excess of calcium or magnesium ions, indicating that the displacement of divalent ions is an important feature of their action.

The tyrocidins are also bactericidal and promote leakage of cytoplasmic solutes. Their action on the bacterial membrane permits passage into the cell of ions that are normally excluded, and under some conditions this causes uncoupling of oxidative phosphorylation as a secondary effect. Gramicidin S, a closely related compound, acts similarly. It lyses protoplasts from *Micrococcus lysodeikticus* but not those from *Bacillus brevis*. Since it is bactericidal towards the former organism but not the latter it is reasonable to suppose that both its action and specificity depend upon its effect on the cytoplasmic membrane. The tyrocidins act not only on bacteria but also on the fungus *Neurospora crassa*. In this organism concentrations of the antibiotic that stop growth and cause leakage of cell contents also cause an immediate fall in membrane potential, a consequence of the destruction of the permeability barrier.

In both the tyrocidin group and in the polymyxins the cyclic structure of the molecule is important for antibacterial activity. The presence of basic groups is also essential, but in other respects the molecules can be varied considerably without losing activity. The simple, symmetrical structure of gramicidin S has been subjected to many modifications. Activity is preserved when the ornithine units are replaced by arginine or lysine groups but is lost by modifications destroying the basic character of the terminal groups. The compound in which glycine replaces L-proline is fully active. Moreover one L-proline residue together with the adjacent D-phenylalanine can be replaced by a δ-aminopentanoic acid group without losing antibacterial activity. The resulting compound has only nine peptide groups, but retains the same ring size. Acyclic compounds having the same sequence of amino acids as gramicidin S show only slight antibacterial action.

The importance of the cyclic structure lies in the maintenance of a well-defined, compact conformation in solution. This has been shown by n.m.r., optical rotary dispersion and other physical measurements. In tyrocidin A and gramicidin S the conformation is determined by lipophilic association between the non-polar side chains of the amino acids, particularly leucine, valine, proline and phenylalanine, and by hydrogen-bonding between the peptide groups. Three regions have been defined in the molecular topography of tyrocidin A: a hydrophobic surface, a flat hydrophilic opposite surface consisting of the peptide groups of most of the amino acids in equatorial positions and a helical hydrophilic region accommodating the amide groups of asparagine and glutamine and the tyrosine hydroxyl group. Gramicidin S shows a similar arrangement, based on a pleated-sheet structure. In both antibiotics the ornithine amino groups, which are essential for antibacterial activity, stand out from the hydrophilic surface.

Cyclosporin A (Fig. 3.4) is an unusual cyclic polypeptide antibiotic in which 7 of the 11 amino acid units are *N*-methylated. It was originally discovered as an antifungal agent, but has proved to have remarkable immunosuppressive properties. Unlike the usual cytotoxic agents it does not cause leucopenia or Cushing's syndrome and it has been used successfully to prevent rejection in organ grafts.

Ionophoric antibiotics

Several classes of antibiotics may be grouped together because of their common property of facilitating the passage of inorganic cations across membranes by formation of hydrophobic complexes. Although these compounds were discovered through their antibacterial activity, they are not used in medicine because of their lack of specificity. They act equally effectively on the membranes of animal cells and may therefore be toxic. Nevertheless they are of considerable biochemical interest and are increasingly used as experimental tools. As antibacterial agents they are active mainly against

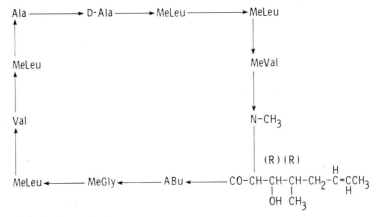

Figure 3.4 Cyclosporin A.

Gram-positive organisms. Gram-negative bacteria are relatively insensitive because their outer membranes are impermeable to hydrophobic compounds of the molecular size of the ionophores. One class of ionophoric antibiotics is typified by valinomycin (Fig. 3.5), the first member of the group to be discovered and the most widely studied. It is a cyclic depsipeptide in which amino acids alternate with hydroxy acids in a ring which contains both peptide and ester groups. An important feature is the alternation of D- and L-configurations in pairs around the 12 components of the ring

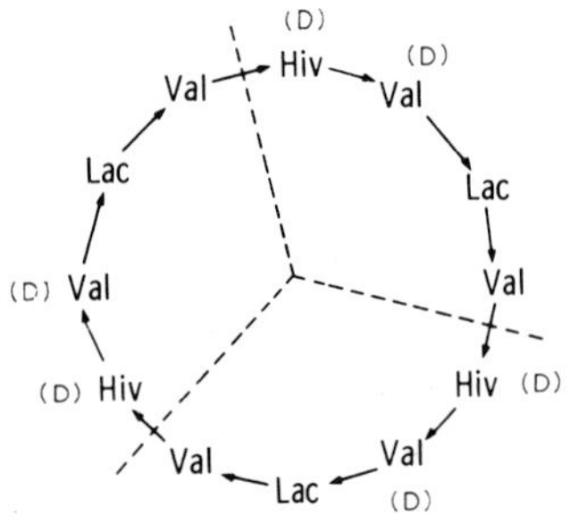

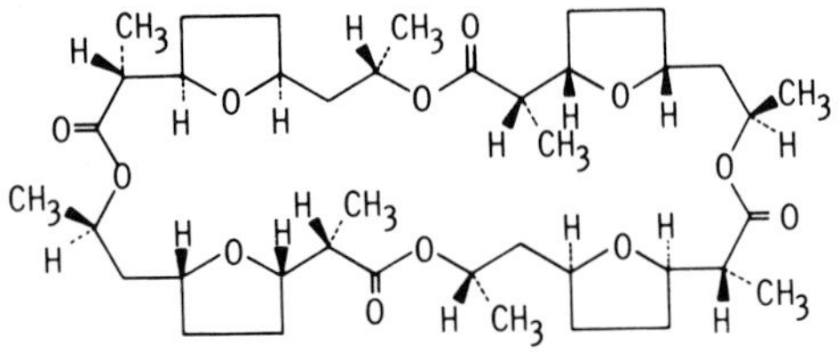

Valinomycin

Nonactin

Figure 3.5 Antibiotics affecting the permeability of membranes to potassium ions. In the valinomycin structure residues are represented thus: Val = valine, Lac = lactic acid, Hiv = 2-hydroxyisovaleric acid. Arrows show the direction of peptide or ester bonds, -CO-NH- or -CO-O-. The asymmetric centres have L-configuration unless otherwise indicated. Dotted lines separate the repeating units.

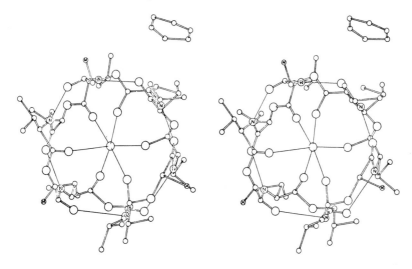

Figure 3.6 Stereophotographs of a model of the potassium complex of valinomycin. To obtain a three-dimensional effect the diagram should be held about 20 inches from the eyes and attention concentrated on the space between the two pictures. With practice three pictures can be seen, the middle one showing a full stereoscopic effect. The central metal ion is seen co-ordinated to six oxygen atoms. Nitrogen atoms are labelled N and the methyl groups of the lactyl residues M. Hydrogen bonds are shown by thin lines. The solitary hexagonal ring is hexane of crystallization. The diagram was generated from X-ray crystallographic data by a computer programme written by Carroll K. Johnson, Oak Ridge, Tennessee. We express our gratitude to Mary Pinkerton and L.K. Steinrauf for supplying this illustration and allowing us to publish it.

structure. This is a common feature of all the cyclic ionophores; where the ring has six components, as in enniatin, the configuration alternates between each component. Valinomycin forms a well-defined complex with potassium ions. This crystalline compound has been studied by X-ray diffraction and shows a highly ordered structure (Fig. 3.6) in which the potassium atom is surrounded by six oxygen atoms. The ring structure is puckered and held in a cylindrical or bracelet-like form by hydrogen bonds roughly parallel to its axis. The ability to achieve such a conformation depends entirely on the alternation of D- and L- centres. The dimensions are such that the potassium atom is exactly accommodated. The ion entering the complex must shed its normal hydration shell; the complex retains the positive charge carried by the ion. The structure observed in the crystal is substantially maintained in solution. Although valinomycin will also form a complex with sodium, the smaller sodium atoms fits much less exactly into the structure and this complex has a stability constant one thousand times smaller than that of the potassium complex.

The high specificity of valinomycin towards the potassium ion and the physical properties of the complex are in accord with its postulated action on biological membranes. In the complex the potassium ion has lost its usual hydration shell and is sheathed instead in a lipophilic envelope built up from the fatty side chains of the amino and hydroxy acids which form the outer surface of the cylinder. Much of the work on valinomycin has been done with artificial membranes, liposomes and mitochondria. In all these the essential action of valinomycin is to facilitate the transport of potassium across the membrane. The lipophilic molecule moves physically through the membrane lipids carrying potassium and returns in the protonated form. In a passive membrane the flow is determined solely by the concentration of potassium ions on each side of the membrane, but in mitochondria supplied with an energy source potassium is taken in by an energy-coupled process against the concentration gradient. The process is highly effective, one valinomycin molecule being able to transport 10^4 ions/s, a turnover rate higher than that of many enzymes. Kinetic studies reveal that the transport of potassium by valinomycin and similar ionophores shows saturation kinetics with respect to the cation; sodium ions inhibit potassium transport although they undergo little transport themselves. The kinetic results are well explained by a model in which the ionophore at the membrane surface first forms a hydrophilic cation complex. This is transformed to a hydrophobic complex which can then cross the membrane. The rate of the transformation from one type of complex to the other determines the turnover number.

The mechanism of the inhibitory action of valinomycin on bacteria has received less study. In the rather simple case of *Streptococcus faecalis* growing anaerobically there is no oxidative phosphorylation mechanism; ATP is generated solely by glycolysis. Valinomycin is inhibitory to this organism in normal media of low potassium content. It specifically drains the cell of potassium and growth ceases because of the requirement for potassium in protein biosynthesis. If the potassium content of the medium is raised to that normally present in the cytoplasm the inhibitory action of valinomycin is prevented. With growing aerobic bacteria the inhibitory action of valinomycin is also a function of its potassium-transporting effect which disturbs oxidative phosphorylation as a secondary consequence.

Another series of antibiotics known as the macrotetrolides

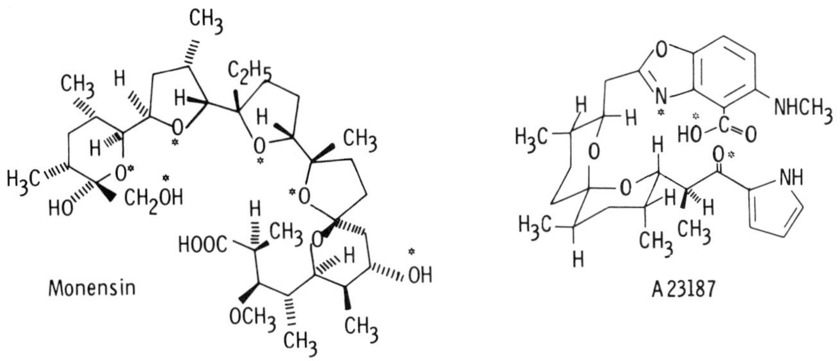

Figure 3.7 Ionophoric antibiotics. For monensin the asterisks show the six oxygen atoms which co-ordinate with the metal ion in the sodium complex. For A23187 the complex with a calcium ion involves two ligand molecules co-ordinated to the metal ion through the atoms marked with an asterisk.

exemplified by nonactin (Fig. 3.5) have a cyclic structure which similarly permits the enclosure of a potassium ion in a cage of eight oxygen atoms (the carbonyl and tetrahydrofuran oxygens), with the rest of the molecule forming an outer lipophilic shell. To produce this structure the ligand is folded in a form resembling the seam of a tennis ball and is held in shape by hydrogen-bonding. The action of the macrotetrolides closely resembles that of valinomycin.

Ionophoric antibiotics of another broad group, typified by monensin (Fig. 3.7) and the closely related nigericin, carry a carboxyl group. In these compounds the molecule itself is not cyclic, but as with valinomycin a metal complex is formed in which the ion is surrounded by ether oxygen atoms and the outer surface is lipophilic. This involves a folding of the molecule which brings the carboxyl group at one end into a position where it can form strong hydrogen bonds with the alcohol groups at the other end; the structure is thus stabilized into an effectively cyclic form. Monensin binds sodium ions preferentially to potassium ions, but in the closely related nigericin, which allows a slightly wider spacing of the oxygen atoms, the selectivity is reversed. The presence of a carboxyl group in these compounds makes an important difference to their action. They promote electrically neutral cation-proton exchange across the membrane by moving as an undissociated acid in one direction and as a cation-anion complex with no net charge in the other direction. This distinguishes them from valinomycin and nonactin where the metal complex carries a positive charge.

These compounds, particularly nigericin, have been studied mainly in artificial membrane and vesicle preparations. They promote a coupled 1:1 exchange of potassium or sodium ions and hydrogen ions. Since no change of charge is involved in complex formation, compounds of this type do not disturb the electrical properties of lipid-bilayer membranes.

Monensin is a compound of considerable commercial importance. It was first introduced as a coccidiostat in chickens, and has proved of exceptional utility. It has shown few signs of the development of resistance which usually terminates the effective life of drugs sold for treating coccidiosis. Later, monensin was found to improve the utilization of feedstuffs in ruminants. Its action depends on altering the balance of free fatty acid production by rumen bacteria in favour of propionate at the expense of acetate. Propionate is energetically more useful to the animal than acetate. There is also a lessening in the metabolically wasteful production of methane. The application of monensin either as a coccidiostat or as a growth promoter was strongly governed by cost and depended on the possibility of producing the compound on a large scale as cheaply as possible. This was successfully achieved by construction of fermentation vessels of unprecedented size. The world usage during 1978 was 1200 tons, and the selling price about £27 per kg. The biochemical basis of the success of monensin in both these applications remains uncertain.

The ionophores considered so far form complexes only with monovalent metal ions. A few ionophores are known which form complexes with divalent ions. Of these perhaps the most interesting is A23187 (Fig. 3.7). This forms a 2:1 complex with calcium or magnesium ions, the calcium complex having the higher stability; it binds monovalent ions only weakly. As with monensin it is not a cyclic molecule but is able to fold into an effectively cyclic conformation by formation of a hydrogen bond between a carboxyl oxygen and the NH group of the pyrrole ring. The divalent metal ion is held in octahedral co-ordination between the polar faces of two ligand molecules. This gives an electrically neutral complex with a hydrophobic outer surface. It acts as a freely mobile carrier of these ions and causes progressive release of magnesium, uncoupling of oxidative phosphorylation and inhibition of adenosine triphosphatase in mitochondria suspended in a magnesium-free medium.

Like monensin, several divalent cationophoric antibiotics can modify rumen fermentation and improve the utilization of feedstuffs by sheep and cattle.

Pore-forming antibiotics

Gramicidin A

Gramicidin A (Fig. 3.8) (quite unrelated to gramicidin S) has many biochemical properties resembling those of valinomycin. It shows a specificity towards potassium ions and promotes their passage across lipid membranes. However, studies have shown that its mechanism of action is different. The most significant demonstration of this distinction depends upon measurements of the electrical conductivity

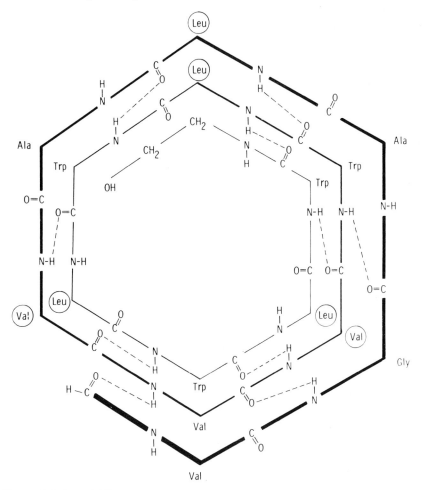

Figure 3.8 Gramicidin A. One possible helical structure having 6.3 residues per turn. Bonds drawn inwards are directed down the helix; those drawn outwards are directed up. D-Amino acid residues are circled.

of artificial membranes separating aqueous layers containing potassium ions. Conditions can be chosen where addition of valinomycin, nonactin or gramicidin A at 0.1 μM concentration lowers the resistance of the membrane at least 1000-fold. If the temperature is now lowered gradually the membrane reaches a transition point at which its lipid layer effectively changes phase from liquid to solid. In the presence of valinomycin or nonactin a $2°C$ fall in temperature at the transition point causes a dramatic rise in membrane resistance, but in a similar experiment with gramicidin A resistance rises only slowly as the temperature falls. The effect with compounds of the valinomycin type is understandable since they require a liquid membrane for mobility and movement. Gramicidin A must act by some process which does not require mobility. The most obvious way is by formation of a pore which would still permit the flow of ions through a rigid membrane. Inspection of the molecular formula of gramicidin A shows it to be a linear polypeptide in which alternating amino acid residues have the L configuration. The remaining residues are either D-amino acids or glycine. The carboxyl terminal is amidated with ethanolamine and the amino terminal carries a formyl group. The configuration allows the molecule to form an open helical structure held together by hydrogen bonds lying almost parallel to the axis of the cylinder. One possible helical form is shown in Fig. 3.8. The inside of the helix is lined with polar groups and there is a central hole about 0.4 nm in diameter. The fatty side chains of the amino acids form a lipophilic shell on the outside. One such molecule is not long enough to form a pore across a membrane, but head to head dimerization is believed to occur by bonds between the formyl groups. The existence of dimerization is supported by measurements in artificial membranes which show that conductance is proportional to the square of the concentration of gramicidin A. The length of the dimer is calculated to be 2.5-3.0 nm which is somewhat less than the thickness of the fatty layer in many membranes so some distortion probably occurs during pore formation.

Conductivity measurements suggest that these pores have a transient existence, a small fraction of the antibiotic being in the form of pores at any given time. The life of a channel measured in a phosphatidylethanolamine artificial membrane was 0.35 s. However, while a pore is in existence, its transporting capacity is high. One channel is estimated to convey 3×10^7 K$^+$ ions/s under a potential gradient of 100 mV. Thus a low concentration of gramicidin A is a very effective carrier of potassium ions.

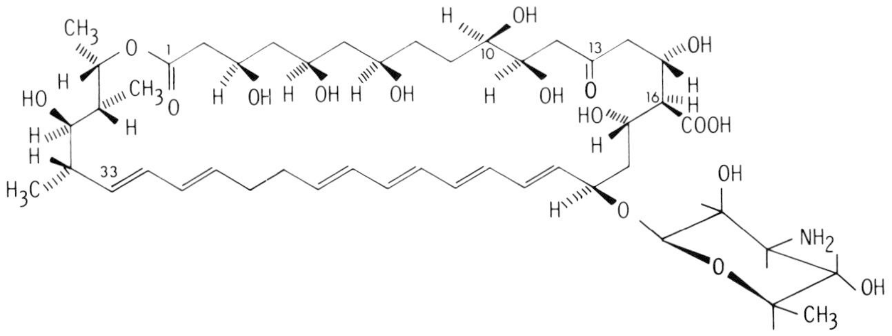

Figure 3.9 Nystatin A_1. Cyclic ketal formation between C_{13} and C_{17} has been demonstrated in the related polyene amphotericin B.

The polyene antibiotics

The polyene antibiotics constitute a large group of varied molecular structure. They are large-ring lactones. Part of the ring is hydrophobic, comprising a sequence of four to seven conjugated double bonds; in another part of the ring many of the carbon atoms bear hydroxyl groups, creating a hydrophilic area. These features can be seen in nystatin (Fig. 3.9). This compound and the closely related amphotericin B are the only polyenes commonly used in medicine. They are active against yeasts and fungi. Although infections by these organisms are rare, they are dangerous when they occur. Amphotericin B given intravenously to treat systemic mycoses invariably causes side effects including kidney damage; but it can halt infections that would otherwise be fatal. The polyenes are not absorbed from the gastrointestinal tract but are sometimes given by mouth to combat fungal growth in the intestine. This most frequently results from the use of broad-spectrum antibiotics which deplete the normal bacterial flora of the gut and allow yeasts and fungi to multiply with troublesome consequences.

The polyene antibiotics act exclusively on cells which have sterols in their cytoplasmic membrane. Thus they affect yeasts, fungi and animal cells but have no effect on most bacteria. Quantitative experiments show that approximately one molecule of polyene antibiotic binds to each sterol molecule in a membrane. Binding can be inhibited by inclusion in the medium of digitonin, a compound known to complex with sterols. The dependence on the presence of sterols for activity is well illustrated by experiments with mycoplasmas, one of the few types of bacteria which sometimes have sterols in their membrane. *Mycoplasma laidlawii* grown on normal media has no sterol in its membrane and is resistant to nystatin. If it is grown instead in a medium containing ergosterol, it incorporates the sterol into its membrane and becomes sensitive to the polyene. *Mycoplasma gallisepticum* which has an absolute requirement for sterols for growth is also sensitive to antibiotics of this class.

Polyenes, in general, bind specifically to sterols having a 3β-hydroxyl group and a relatively long side chain. Many of them bind readily to cholesterol and are consequently very toxic to animal cells. The larger polyenes, nystatin and amphotericin B, show a preferred interaction with 3β-hydroxy sterols, having a conjugated diene in the nucleus. This confers some selective action against the fungi, which normally contain ergosterol, compared with erythrocytes and other body cells which have cholesterol in their membranes. They can therefore be used systemically in fungal infections, but their interaction with cholesterol is still sufficient to cause problems of haemolysis and nephritis.

The action of compounds of this group is to increase the permeability of the fungal membrane. This is shown by their ability to cause leakage of intracellular solutes. Work with fungal cells, erythrocytes and vesicles containing sterols has shown that nystatin and amphotericin alter membrane permeability so as to allow ready passage of sodium and potassium ions, and small molecules up to the size of glucose. Conductivity measurements with artificial membranes indicate that the permeability effects clearly result from the formation of pores across the membrane. Attempts have been made to link these observations with the structure of the polyenes.

Molecular models of amphotericin B and nystatin show a rod-like structure held rigid by the all-*trans* extended conjugated system which is equal in length to an ergosterol molecule. The cross-section of the polyene structure is roughly rectangular. One surface of the rod is hydrophobic and the opposite surface, studded with axial hydroxyl groups, is hydrophilic. At one end of the rod the mycosamine sugar group and the carboxyl group form a zwitterionic assembly with strongly polar properties. In models it is possible to assemble about 10 molecules of amphotericin B with their long axes parallel to form a cylinder. This has the hydrophilic groups on the inside and the hydrophobic groups on the outside, with one sterol molecule tucked in between each pair of molecules on the hydrophobic surface. This would constitute a pore of the correct internal diameter (0.7 nm) having a length equal to half the width of the membrane. Such a structure would accommodate itself in the membrane with the polar head group at the surface and the lipophilic outer cylinder in the lipid interior. Two such structures end to end would span the membrane and provide the observed permeability.

The idea is speculative. It provides an explanation of the known facts, but requires experimental verification. The polyenes certainly form pores, and this formation is dependent on the presence of sterols. As with gramicidin A, the pores need only be transient, involving a small proportion of the polyene and sterol molecules at any one time.

Further reading

General
P.A. LAMBERT (1978), 'Membrane-active antimicrobial agents', in *Prog. Med. Chem.*, 15, 88.
W.B. HUGO (1978), 'Membrane-active antimicrobial drugs - a reappraisal of their mode of action in the light of the chemiosmotic theory', in *Int. J. Pharmaceut.*, 1, 127.
M.R.J. SALTON and P. OWEN (1976), 'Bacterial membrane structure', in *Annu. Rev. Microbiol.*, 30, 451.
W.A. HAMILTON (1974), 'Recent research on the action of antibiotics on microbial membranes', in *Industrial Aspects of Biochemistry*, ed. B. Spencer, FEBS (North-Holland, 1974).
M.R.J. SALTON and A. TOMASZ (eds) (1974), 'Mode of action of antibiotics on microbial walls and membrane' *in Anna. N.Y. Acad. Sci.*, 235, (1974).

Antiseptics and disinfectants
B. LYNN (1977), 'Chemical disinfectants, antiseptics and preservatives', in *Pharmaceutical Microbiology*, p. 155, ed. W.B. Hugo and J.B. Russell, (Blackwell, 1977).
W.B. HUGO (1977), 'Mode of action of non-antibiotic antimicrobial agents', in *Pharmaceutical Microbiology*, p. 202, ed. W.B. Hugo and J.B. Russell, (Blackwell, 1977).
W.B. HUGO (1976), 'The inactivation of vegetative bacteria by chemicals', in *The Inactivation of Vegetative Bacteria*, Symposium: Society of Applied Bacteriology, ed. F.A. Skinner and W.B. Hugo, (Academic Press, 1976).

Polypeptide antibiotics
D.R. STORM, K.S. ROSENTHAL and P.E. SWANSON (1977), 'Polymyxin and related peptide antibiotics', in *Annu. Rev. Biochem.*, 46, 723.
Y.A. OVCHINNIKOV and V.T. IVANOV (1975), 'Conformational states and biological activity of cyclic peptides', in *Tetrahedron*, 31, 2177.
JUN'ICHI SHOJI (1978), 'Recent chemical studies on peptide antibiotics from the genus *Bacillus*', in *Adv. Appl. Microbiol.*, 24, 187.

Ionophoric antibiotics
P.W. REED (1979), 'Ionophores' in *Methods Enzymol.*, 55, 435.
E.P. BAKKER (1979), 'Ionophore antibiotics', in *Antibiotics*, Vol. 5 Part 2, p. 67, ed. F.E. Hahn, (Springer Verlag, 1979).

Polyene antibiotics

R.W. HOLZ (1979), 'Polyene antibiotics: nystatin, amphotericin B and filipin', in *Antibiotics*, Vol. 5, Part 2, p. 313, ed. F.E. Hahn, (Springer Verlag, 1979).
S.M. HAMMOND (1977), 'Biological activity of polyene antibiotics', in *Prog. Med. Chem.*, 14, 106.
A.W. NORMAN, A.M. SPIELVOGEL and R.G. WONG (1976), 'Polyene antibiotic-sterol interaction', in *Adv. Lipid Res.*, 14, 127.

4 Suppression of gene function 1.
Inhibitors of the synthesis
of nucleic acids

Many antimicrobial substances, both synthetic chemicals and natural products, directly inhibit the biosynthesis of nucleic acids. However, very few of these inhibitors have found clinical use as antimicrobial drugs because most of them do not distinguish between the nucleic acid synthesis by the infecting micro-organism and that by the host. Usually, therefore, inhibitors of nucleic acid synthesis are too toxic to the host animal for safe use as antimicrobial agents. However, there are a few exceptions to this rule which are described in this chapter. Some inhibitors of nucleic acid synthesis are used as anticancer agents, although their administration to patients is fraught with danger because of their lack of selectivity between normal and neoplastic cells. Not only are the dividing cancer cells attacked but also the rapidly dividing normal cells of the body. Strictly speaking, anticancer drugs fall outside the scope of this book. However, since several of these drugs have interesting effects on nucleic acid synthesis, a few examples are given to illustrate different modes of attack both on the biosynthesis of nucleic acid precursors and on the polymerization process.

The synthesis of DNA and the various classes of RNA is an essential function of dividing and growing cells. Thus inhibition of DNA synthesis rapidly results in inhibition of cell division. In addition, the biosynthesis and intercellular exchange of extra-chromosomal elements of DNA in bacteria, the episomes and plasmids, are important in maintaining the flexible responses of bacteria to changes in the environment (Chapter 8).

The inhibition of RNA synthesis is followed by cessation of protein synthesis. The time elapsing between the inhibition of RNA synthesis induced by a drug such as actinomycin D and the resulting failure of protein biosynthesis may be used to indicate the rate of utilization and destruction of messenger RNA in intact cells.

Types of inhibitors of nucleic acid synthesis

Substances which inhibit nucleic acid synthesis fall into two main categories. One group includes compounds that interfere with the elaboration of the 'building blocks' of nucleic acids, that is the purine and pyrimidine nucleotides. Interruption of the synthesis of any one of the nucleoside triphosphates required for nucleic acid synthesis stops further macromolecular synthesis when the nucleotide precursor pool has been exhausted. This group includes many structural analogues of purines and pyrimidines and their respective nucleosides. Few, if any, of such compounds have been useful as antibacterial drugs because of their lack of specificity. However, a number of purine and pyrimidine analogues that have been used as anticancer and antiviral drugs are described later. Drugs that interfere with the biosynthesis of folic acid referred to in Chapter 6 are powerful indirect inhibitors of nucleotide biosynthesis. Tetrahydrofolate acts as a donor of one-carbon units in several steps in purine and pyrimidine nucleotide biosynthesis. Interruption of the supply of tetrahydrofolate by antifolate drugs soon brings nucleotide and nucleic acid synthesis to a halt. Some of the antifolate drugs show considerable species specificity and are therefore valuable as antimicrobial agents (Chapter 6).

The other group of inhibitors interferes with nucleic acid synthesis at the polymerization stage. This type of inhibition is often due to an interaction between the inhibitor and DNA and may prevent either the replication of DNA itself or interfere with the template function of DNA in RNA synthesis. Other inhibitors of polymerization hinder the function of the polymerases by direct interaction with these enzymes or the enzyme-template complexes. As we shall see, polymerase inhibitors often exhibit species specificity.

Inhibitors of the biosynthesis of nucleotide precursors

Many inhibitors of the synthesis of nucleotide precursors block the elaboration of purine nucleotides. The complex series of reactions leading to the formation of adenine and guanine nucleoside monophosphates is summarized in Fig. 4.1. We shall refer only to those steps that are relevant to the mode of action of the inhibitors.

Azaserine and 6-diazo-5-oxo-L-norleucine (DON)

Both these antibiotics are produced by streptomycetes and they are structurally quite similar. They may be regarded as analogues of

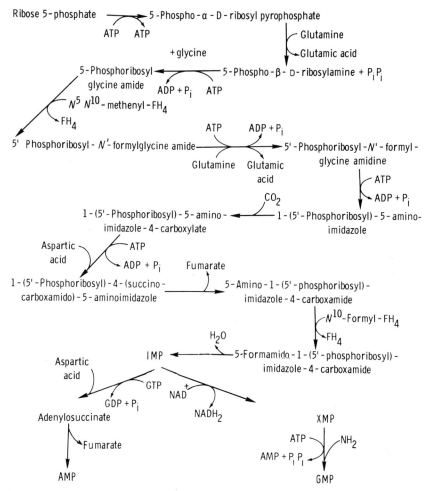

Figure 4.1 Reaction sequence leading to the biosynthesis of adenine and guanine nucleotides. P_i and P_iP_i indicate inorganic phosphate and pyrophosphate respectively and FH_4 indicates tetrahydrofolic acid. The amino group involved in the conversion of XMP into GMP is derived from ammonia in bacteria but from glutamine in mamallian cells.

glutamine (Fig. 4.2). Azaserine and DON inhibit the growth of many micro-organisms, but because they are also toxic to mammalian cells they have only been used clinically as antitumour drugs.

Both drugs prevent the attachment of glutamine to its binding site on the enzyme which converts formylglycine amide ribonucleotide to the corresponding amidine. Azaserine combines irreversibly with the SH group the active centre. DON reacts similarly with the SH

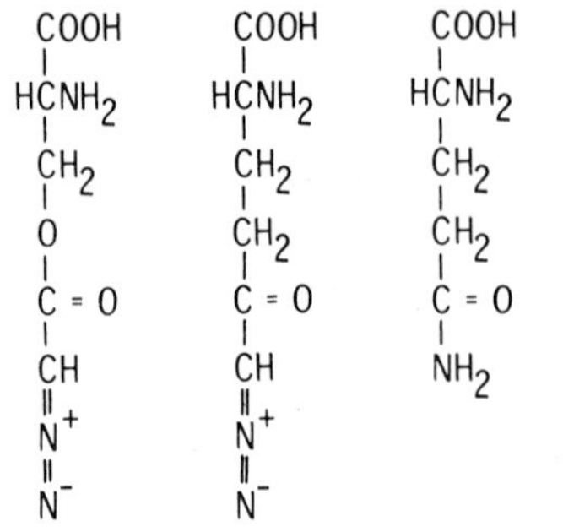

```
   COOH        COOH        COOH
    |           |           |
  HCNH2       HCNH2       HCNH2
    |           |           |
   CH2         CH2         CH2
    |           |           |
    O          CH2         CH2
    |           |           |
   C = 0       C = 0       C = 0
    |           |           |
   CH          CH          NH2
   ‖ +         ‖ +
   N           N
   ‖ −         ‖ −
   N           N
```

Azaserine   'DON'   Glutamine

Figure 4.2 The structural similarities between the antibiotics azaserine and diazo-oxonorleucine ('DON') and the amino acid glutamine can be seen in this diagram.

group at the glutamine-binding site of cytidine triphosphate synthetase, the enzyme that catalyses the transfer of an -NH$_2$ group from glutamine to UTP. Despite the similarities between azaserine and DON, there are also important differences. For example, DON is more potent than azaserine as an inhibitor of purine nucleotide biosynthesis, while azaserine has radiomimetic and mutagenic properties that are lacking in DON.

Hadacidin

A product of many species of *Penicillium*, hadacidin (*N*-formyl-hydroxyaminoacetic acid) is an analogue and antagonist of L-aspartic acid (Fig. 4.3). Hadacidin has both antimicrobial and anticancer activity, although its clinical effectiveness against human malignant disease is disappointing.

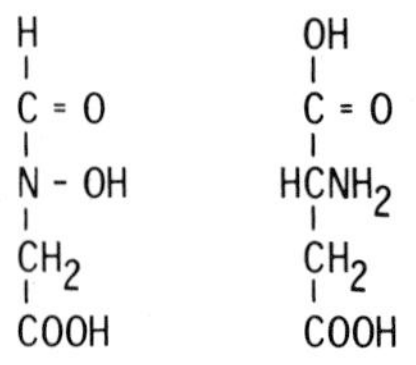

```
    H            OH
    |            |
   C = 0        C = 0
    |            |
   N - OH      HCNH2
    |            |
   CH2          CH2
    |            |
   COOH         COOH
```

Hadacidin   L - Aspartic acid

Figure 4.3 Hadacidin, an antibiotic resembling L-aspartic acid.

Hadacidin inhibits the conversion of IMP in mammalian cells to adenylosuccinic acid, and the inhibition is partially reversed by L-aspartic acid. Purified adenylosuccinate synthetase from *Escherichia coli* is also competitively inhibited by hadacidin. The K'_m for L-aspartate is $150\mu M$ (pH8.0), while the K_i for hadacidin is $4.2\mu M$. Hadacidin is thus an effective competitive antagonist of L-aspartate in the conversion of IMP to adenylosuccinic acid. It is therefore surprising to find that hadacidin has little or no antagonistic activity against L-aspartate in other reactions involving this amino acid. For example, the conversion of 1-(5'-phosphoribosyl)-5-aminoimidazole-4-carboxylate to the corresponding amide which also requires L-aspartate is not affected by hadacidin. Again, hadacidin only very weakly competes with L-aspartate in pyrimidine biosynthesis and has no direct effect on protein biosynthesis. Apparently hadacidin only significantly hinders the substrate functions of L-aspartate under the specific conditions of the amidation of IMP. At present we have no molecular explanation of this interesting specificity.

Psicofuranine and decoyinine

Psicofuranine is a naturally occurring antibiotic (from *Streptomyces hygroscopicus* var. *decoyicus*) with a nucleoside type of structure (Fig. 4.4). It has both antimicrobial and anticancer activity. However, its use as an anticancer drug has been limited by a tendency to cause pericarditis in man.

Despite its structural resemblance to adenosine, psicofuranine inhibits nucleic acid synthesis in bacteria by blocking the final stage in the biosynthesis of GMP, i.e. the amination of XMP. The enzyme that catalyses this reaction in *E. coli* is inhibited non-competitively by psicofuranine and also by the closely related antibiotic decoyinine (Fig. 4.4). This inhibition is reversed by adenosine, which itself may inhibit XMP aminase non-competitively. The inhibition by psicofuranine, however, is not reversed by either xanthosine or guanosine. Certain reagents, such as urea and 2-mercaptoethanol, 'desensitize' XMP aminase to the action of psicofuranine and decoyinine and yet preserve the catalytic function of the enzyme. This suggests that these antibiotics do not act at the active site of the enzyme but at an allosteric site that provides an inhibitory control mechanism in the native enzyme. Desensitization may modify the allosteric site so that it no longer binds the inhibitory nucleoside derivatives. The inhibition of XMP aminase by adenosine presumably fulfils some control function in purine nucleotide metabolism.

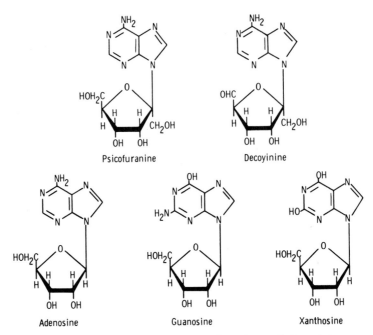

Figure 4.4 Two nucleoside antibiotics, psicofuranine and decoyinine compared with normal purine nucleosides.

Mycophenolic acid

This is an antibiotic of considerable antiquity which was first detected in 1896 as a product of *Penicillium stoloniferum*. Chemical studies eventually revealed its chemical structure some 50 years later (Fig. 4.5). The antibacterial activity of mycophenolic acid is very limited, although its activity against a range of fungi is more striking. It also has excellent activity against many experimental tumours in rodents. Unfortunately the compound proved to be inactive against human cancers, apparently because it is rapidly metabolized in man to an inactive product.

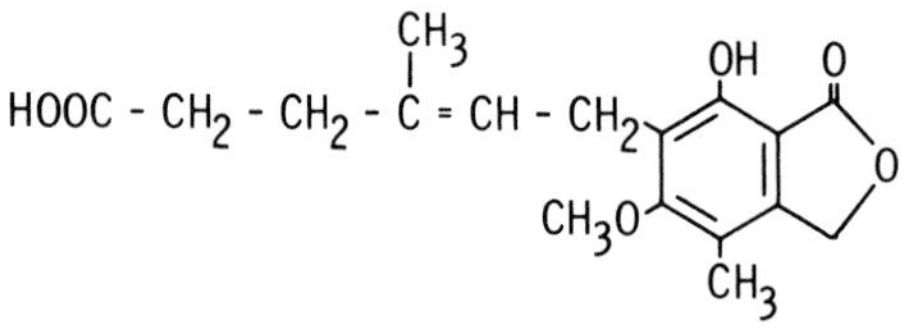

Figure 4.5 Mycophenolic acid.

The antimitotic action of the antibiotic depends mainly on its inhibition of the enzyme which converts IMP to XMP, i.e. IMP dehydrogenase (IMP-NAD$^+$ oxidoreductase). This rapidly arrests the supply of guanine nucleotides essential for DNA and RNA synthesis. All the inhibitors described so far in this chapter are structural analogues and antagonists of the natural intermediates in the biosynthesis of purine nucleotides. With mycophenolic acid, however, it is difficult to see any significant structural resemblance to IMP or NAD$^+$ or indeed to any other reactant in purine nucleotide metabolism. Mycophenolic acid may conceivably induce conformational distortions in the enzyme that hinder its normal functioning, although direct experimental evidence for this is lacking. Prolonged storage of a preparation of IMP dehydrogenase from *Bacillus subtilis* leads to a partial loss of sensitivity of the enzyme to mycophenolic acid, suggesting that the inhibitor does not act directly at the active site but may exert a more subtle form of control over the enzyme.

Inhibitors of nucleic acid synthesis at the polymerization level

In the final stage of nucleic acid synthesis the nucleoside triphosphates are condensed into a polynucleotide chain in which the constituent nucleosides are joined by 3′-5′-phosphodiester linkages; inorganic phosphate is formed during the polymerization. The nucleoside triphosphates react sequentially under the influence of the appropriate polymerase. The biosynthesis of the polynucleotide proceeds in a 5′ to 3′ direction. The sequence in which the nucleotides are added is, of course, governed strictly by the base-pairing requirements of the template strand. In DNA synthesis, the initiation of the new strand also requires a primer, i.e. a strand terminating in a free 3′-OH group on which the first nucleotide can substitute. RNA synthesis on the other hand does not require a primer for strand initiation. During the replication of double-helical DNA both strands are copied simultaneously in an antiparallel manner. In RNA synthesis, however, only the so-called 'plus' strand of the DNA acts as a template.

Inhibitors of polynucleotide chain formation act either by disturbing the template function of the nucleic acid or by direct inhibition of the specific polymerase. Substances that disturb template function always interact in some way with the nucleic acid. This inhibitor-nucleic acid interaction usually causes profound changes in the physical properties of the macromolecule. While inhibition of polymerase function may be an indirect result of the interaction between the inhibitor and the template molecule, inhibition of polymerase activity can also result from a direct attack of the inhibitor on the enzyme or on the specific subcellular location of the template-enzyme complex. In bacteria, at least, the subcellular site for DNA replication is thought to be on the cytoplasmic membrane.

A. Intercalating compounds

Many rigidly planar, polycyclic molecules interact with double-helical DNA by a mechanism known as intercalation. The planar character of such molecules enables them to insert or intercalate between the adjacent stacked base-pairs of the double helix. To permit this insertion, there must be a preliminary local unwinding of the double helix to produce spaces between the stacked pairs into which the planar polycyclic molecule can move. The much reproduced diagram in Fig. 4.6 shows schematically how polycyclic structures may intercalate between the stacked base-pairs. The hydrogen-bonding between the base-pairs remains undisturbed, although there is some distortion of the smooth coil of the sugar phosphate backbone as the intercalated molecules maintain the double helix in a partially unwound configuration.

The details of a specific drug-DNA interaction depend largely on the structure of the drug, and several examples are described below. The intercalation of a molecule into DNA is detectable by various physical changes. DNA solutions show an increase in viscosity; there is a decrease in sedimentation coefficient and an increase in thermal stability. The extent of these changes is proportional to the amount of drug intercalated into the double helix.

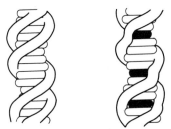

Figure 4.6 These diagrams represent the secondary structure of normal DNA (left) and DNA containing intercalated molecules (right); the stacked bases are separated at intervals by the intercalated molecules resulting in some distortion of the sugar phosphate backbone of the DNA. This diagram is reproduced by kind permission of Dr L. Lerman and the Wistar Press. [*J. Cell. Comp. Physiol.*, **64**, Supplement 1 (1964 I)].

The increase in the viscosity of DNA solutions treated with inter-calating drugs is explained by the restricted degree of irregular tertiary coiling that the double helix can undergo. The DNA-drug complex is, therefore, both straighter and stiffer than the uncomplexed nucleic acid and these changes raise the viscosity. The reductions in sedimentation coefficient and buoyant density of DNA following intercalation result from a reduction in the mass per unit length of the nucleic acid. For example, a proflavine molecule (Fig. 4.7) increases the length of the DNA by about the same amount as an extra base-pair, but because proflavine has less than half the mass of the base-pair, the mass per unit length of the complexed DNA is decreased. The increased thermal stability of intercalated DNA is probably due in part to the extra energy needed to remove the bound molecule from the double helix in addition to that required to separate the strands. Undoubtedly, electrostatic interactions between the intercalated molecule and the two DNA strands assist stabilization of the double helix.

In certain tumour viruses and bacteriophages, in the kinetoplasts of trypanosomes and in bacteria harbouring sex factors and drug-resistance factors (see Chapter 8) double-stranded DNA exists as covalently closed circles. Isolated, circular DNA that is covalently closed via the usual 3'-5'-phosphodiester bond is characteristically supercoiled. These supercoils occur because the circular molecule is in a state of strain. The strain is relieved and the supercoils often disappear when single-stranded breaks or 'nicks' are produced by the action of an endonuclease. Closed circular DNA has an unusual affinity for intercalating molecules which, because they partially unwind the double helix, also reduce the supercoiling of the DNA. If the unwinding proceeds beyond a certain point, as more and more drug is added, the DNA starts to adopt the supercoiled form again, except that the supercoiling occurs in the opposite direction from that of the uncomplexed DNA. At this point the affinity of the closed circuit DNA for the intercalated molecules actually declines until it is less than that of nicked DNA.

The diminished affinity of closed circular DNA for ethidium (Fig. 4.7) at   high concentrations of the drug permits a convenient separation of closed circular DNA from nicked DNA, as the sedimentation coefficient and buoyant density of DNA with a lower content of intercalated material is significantly higher. This effect has been invaluable in the isolation of closed circular DNA on a preparative scale.

It is also possible that the initial higher affinity of supercoiled DNA for intercalating molecules may in part account for their

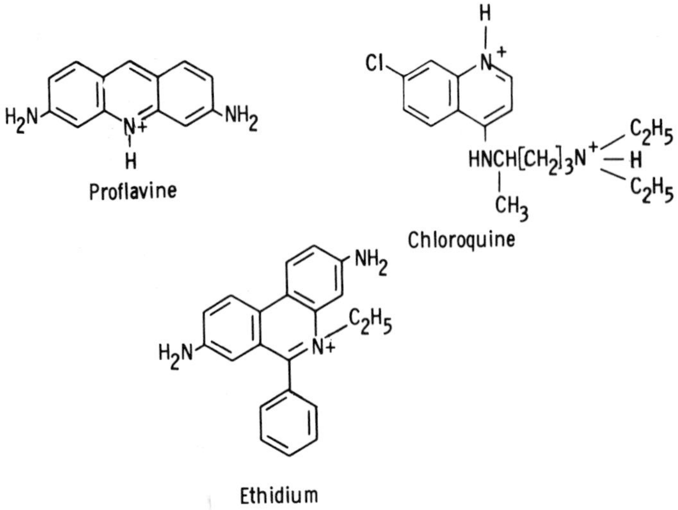

Figure 4.7 Three molecules that intercalate with DNA.

peculiar specificity of action against organelles and organisms believed to contain circular DNA. Extrachromosomal genetic elements in bacteria known as plasmids (Chapter 8) occur to a considerable extent as closed circular DNA. Treatment with acridines under the appropriate conditions of bacteria harbouring plasmids may lead to the disappearance of the plasmids from the cells. While a complete explanation of this phenomenon is lacking, it is possible that preferential interaction of the closed circuit DNA with acridine may be involved. The mitochondria of certain strains of yeast are severely and irreversibly damaged by growth in the presence of ethidium apparently owing to a drug-induced cytoplasmic mutation affecting the mitochondrial DNA. The kinetoplast of trypanosomes is also seriously affected by intercalating agents, DNA synthesis in this organelle being selectively inhibited. Eventually the kinetoplast disappears altogether. As this adversely affects the life cycle of trypanosomes it is possible that the selective attack on the kineto-plast may underlie the trypanocidal activity of certain intercalating drugs.

Acridines, phenanthridines and chloroquine

The medical history of the acridine dyes extends over some 60 years since proflavine (Fig. 4.7) was used as a topical disinfectant on wounds during the First World War. Proflavine is too toxic to be used as a systemic antibacterial agent, but the related acridine, mepacrine (Fig. 1.2), found wide application as an antimalarial drug. Chloroquine (Fig. 4.7) is still an important antimalarial agent and the phenanthridine compound ethidium (Fig. 4.7) is a useful trypanocide.

The compounds all bind to the nucleic acids of living cells and the phenomenon forms the basis of vital staining, since the nucleic acid-dye complexes exhibit characteristic colours when examined by fluorescence microscopy. The dyes also bind readily to nucleic acids *in vitro* and the visible absorption spectra of the ligand molecules undergo a metachromatic shift to longer wavelengths. Two types of binding with DNA are recognized; a strong primary binding and weak secondary binding. The strong primary binding occurs only with DNA, although many other polymers bind the dyes by the secondary process. Primary binding to DNA, which is mainly responsible for the ability of these drugs to interfere with nucleic acid synthesis, causes changes characteristic of intercalation. The location of the intercalated molecule may be stabilized by electronic interaction between its fused rings and the heterocyclic bases of the DNA above and below it. The complex may also be stabilized by hydrogen-bonding between the amino groups of the proflavine and ethidium and the charged oxygen atoms of the phosphate groups in the sugar phosphate backbone. In the case of chloroquine the projecting cationic side chain may form a salt linkage with the phosphate residue.

Actinomycin D

This complex antibiotic (Fig. 4.8) was discovered in 1940. It is an exceedingly toxic substance and consequently has no therapeutic value as an antimicrobial agent. The main interest in actinomycin D lies in its unique interaction with DNA and its application as a specific

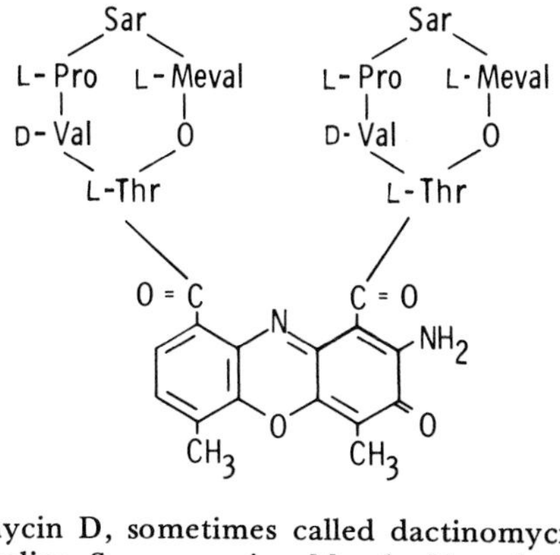

Figure 4.8 Actinomycin D, sometimes called dactinomycin. Thr = threonine, Val = valine, Pro = proline, Sar = sarcosine, Meval = *N*-methylvaline.

inhibitor of DNA-dependent RNA synthesis in cell biology. Actinomycin D also has a limited clinical use as an anticancer agent particularly in the treatment of a renal tumour of children known as Wilm's tumour.

The interaction between DNA and actinomycin D is readily demonstrated: addition of DNA causes a prompt change in the absorption spectrum of actinomycin D solutions. The addition of RNA, however, has no such effect. Furthermore, addition of DNA to solutions of biologically inactive derivatives of actinomycin D does not change their spectra. The following structural features of the actinomycin D molecule are involved in the interaction with DNA: (i) The intact, cyclic pentapeptide lactones are indispensible. Both in solutions of actinomycin and in crystalline complexes of the drug with deoxyguanosine and oligonucleotides, the peptidilactones extend laterally from the tricyclic chromophore, rather like the arms of the letter T (Fig. 4.9). The amino acid sequence is apparently not critical, although replacement of the L-*N*-methyl valine with L-valine abolishes the ability to interact with DNA. (ii) Monomethylation of the amino group of the chromophore causes a 90 per cent loss of activity; other substitutions or removal of the amino group abolish activity entirely. (iii). The quinonoid oxygen is also essential for activity.

The DNA must also have certain essential features for it to interact with actinomycin D: (i) The DNA must contain guanine, although the related base 2, 6-diaminopurine can substitute for guanine in synthetic DNA polymers. (ii) The DNA must be a double-stranded, helical structure. The small degree of binding that occurs between actinomycin D and heat-denatured DNA is probably due to limited helical regions formed as the DNA is rapidly cooled. (iii) The sugar moiety must be deoxyribose; double-stranded RNA (containing guanine) does not interact with actinomycin D to any significant extent.

Intercalations of actinomycin D

The planar character of the chromophoric ring of the drug suggested that its interaction with DNA might involve intercalation. This is supported by the observation that the viscosity of solutions of low-molecular-weight DNA is increased by the addition of actinomycin D, although curiously the drug has the opposite effect on solutions of high-molecular-weight DNA. Another important indication that actinomycin D intercalates with DNA is that the drug first removes and then reverses the supercoils of closed, circular double-stranded DNA. Finally, actinomycin D causes a marked fall in the buoyant

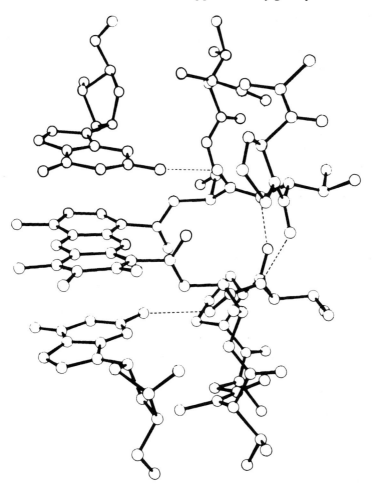

Figure 4.9 Computer-drawn illustration derived from the X-ray crystallographic analysis of the complex of one molecule of actinomycin D with two molecules of deoxyguanosine. The complex is viewed from one side and the chromophore of actinomycin D can be seen sandwiched between the two purine rings. The dotted lines represent the hydrogen bonds which link the pentapeptide rings of the antibiotic to each other and those which link the guanine 2-amino groups with the carbonyl oxygens of the L-threonine residues of the antibiotic. Additional, weaker H-bonds, which are not shown, are also proposed between th guanine N_3-ring nitrogens and the NH groups of the L-threonines. The diagram is reproduced with the kind permission of Dr. H.M. Sobell and the Editors of 'Nature New Biology' [*Nature (London) New Biol.* (1971), **231**, 200].

density of DNA and a striking increase in its thermal stability.

Detailed X-ray studies of a crystalline complex formed between one molecule of actinomycin D and two molecules of deoxyguanosine have revealed that the guanine residues are stacked above and below the chromophoric ring of actinomycin D (Fig. 4.9). The drug molecule is stabilized internally by hydrogen-bonding between its two cyclic pentapeptides; two hydrogen bonds are formed between the NH of the D-valine in one ring and the CO of the D-valine in the other ring. The two cyclic pentapeptides are thus held in such a way that strong hydrogen-bonding can occur between the 2-amino groups of the guanine residues and the CO groups of the L-threonines. Weaker hydrogen bonds connect the ring nitrogen in the 3-position of the guanines with the NH groups on the same L-threonines. Hydrophobic bonding is also thought to occur between the deoxyribose residues and the isopropyl groups of the N-methyl valines.

Extending this model to the complex between actinomycin D and DNA, the cyclic pentapeptides are thought to lie in the minor groove of the double helix. Additional hydrogen-bonding could occur between the 2-amino group of the drug chromophore and a phosphate oxygen and also the sugar-ring oxygen of a deoxycytidine residue. (Remember, of course, that in a duplex DNA molecule the guanine residues stacked above and below actinomycin D would be base-paired with cytosine residues.)

Bifunctional intercalating drugs: the quinoxaline antibiotics

The quinoxaline antibiotics are complex molecules exemplified by echinomycin and triostin A (Fig. 4.10) which are produced by several streptomycetes. They are powerfully cytotoxic molecules, active against Gram-positive bacteria but not against Gram-negative organisms probably because they fail to penetrate the outer envelope. Since they are very toxic to dividing mammalian cells, the quinoxalines have some limited use as experimental anticancer agents in man. Their cytotoxic action has been traced to their interaction with DNA. The binding of each echinomycin molecule extends the double helix by 0.63 nm, which is almost twice the distance that accomodates a single intercalated aromatic chromophore.

This extension is explained if echinomycin intercalates both of its quinoxaline rings into DNA. The other physical changes in DNA molecules brought about by interaction with echinomycin, i.e. reduction in sedimentation coefficient, removal and reversal of super-coiling, are also consistent with intercalation. The peptide ring of echinomycin is rigid and quite planar and the whole molecule can be

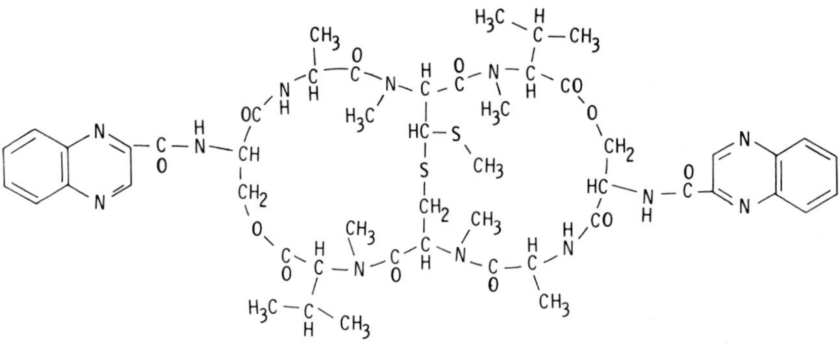

Echinomycin

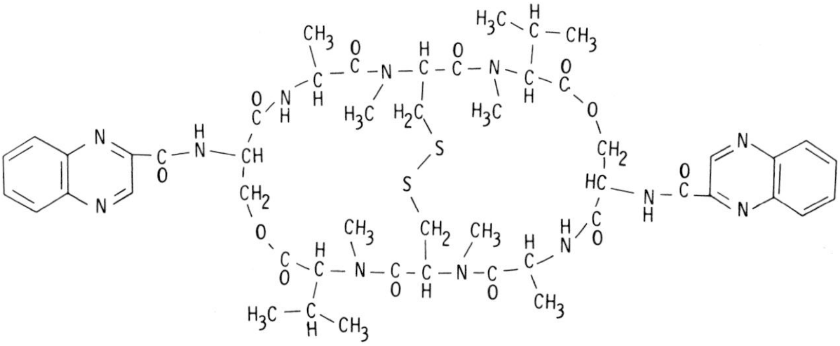

Triostin A

Figure 4.10 Two quinoxaline antibiotics: echinomycin and triostin A.

considered as a rigid disc with the planar quinoxaline rings at opposite ends extending in the same direction perpendicular to the plane of the disc. This unique structure enables the insertion of the twin quinoxaline residues into the double helix at locations approximately 1 nm, i.e. two DNA base-pairs, apart. The integrity of the octapeptide ring must be essential for intercalation because the dimethyl ester of echinomycinic acid, in which the ring is ruptured, cannot interact with DNA. An intact cross-bridge in the peptide ring is also essential, though it can vary in length and constitution, as exemplified in triostin A (Fig. 4.10) which is as potent as echinomycin as a bifunctional intercalater. Nevertheless the nature of the cross-bridge does influence the ability to recognize certain co-polymers. Triostin, for example, binds more effectively to poly[d(A-T)] than to poly[d(G-C)] whereas the reverse is true for echinomycin.

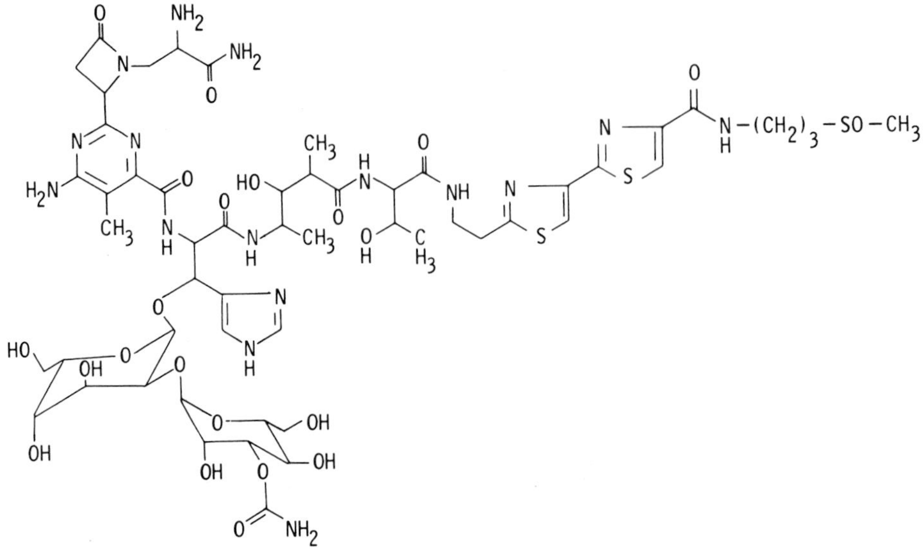

Bleomycin A$_1$

Figure 4.11 Bleomycin A$_1$: a member of a closely related family of antibiotics that 'catalyse' the breakage of DNA chains.

Bleomycins: DNA-strand-breaking drugs that may intercalate

The bleomycins comprise a family of complex, closely related antibiotics (Fig. 4.11). These compounds are toxic to mammalian cells as well as to Gram-positive bacteria and so their medicinal use is confined to anticancer treatment. We describe them here because their biochemical action on DNA is unique.

The bleomycins produce single- and double-stranded breaks in DNA molecules and release the DNA bases. Ferrous iron, which forms a tight complex with bleomycin, molecular oxygen and magnesium ions are required for the strand-breaking reaction. This reaction resembles a catalytic process, since the bleomycin molecule is used repeatedly to produce chain scissions. The chemical mechanism of the action of bleomycins on DNA is uncertain but the first step may involve partial intercalation of the bis-thiazole ring system, possibly adjacent to thymine. Since the strand-breaking action of bleomycin would normally obscure the characteristic changes caused by intercalation, experiments were specially designed to minimize strand breakage. It could then be shown that bleomycin relaxes the supercoils of closed circular DNA and that linear DNA is lengthened by 0.31 nm by each intercalating molecule of bleomycin. The attached bleomycin can then degrade DNA by a reaction which is thought to involve the conversion of the complexed Fe(II) to Fe(III) and the release of either hydroxyl radicals or superoxide anions, which bring about the elimination of the neighbouring thymine residue and eventually scission of the DNA chains.

Inhibition of nucleic acid synthesis by intercalating drugs

The intercalating compounds inhibit both DNA synthesis and DNA-dependent RNA synthesis in intact cells and in cell-free preparations. Some compounds such as actinomycin D and ethidium inhibit RNA synthesis at drug concentrations much lower than those needed to inhibit DNA synthesis. Others such as proflavine interfere equally with DNA or RNA synthesis. Since strand separation is an essential for replication of DNA, the increased stability of the double helix following intercalation may be a major factor in the inhibition of DNA replication. In the inhibition of DNA-dependent RNA synthesis, the intercalated molecules probably hinder the attachment of RNA polymerase to the DNA template so that the number of initiations of new RNA molecules is markedly decreased. The elongation of the nucleic acid chain is also inhibited by the presence of intercalated molecules in the template.

One possible explanation for the selective action of actinomycin D against RNA synthesis is that the RNA polymerase finds its normal progression along the minor groove blocked by the presence of the cyclic pentapeptide rings. The inhibition of DNA synthesis caused by higher concentrations of actinomycin D may be associated with the greater stability of the double helix brought about by an increased number of drug molecules bound to the DNA. The strand-breaking bleomycins are so destructive to the DNA template that both DNA and RNA synthesis rapidly fail after drug treatment.

B. Cross-linkers of DNA: mitomycin and porfiromycin

Mitomycin C and porfiromycin (Fig. 4.12) belong to a series of chemically related substances that are produced by various species of streptomycetes. They are powerful antimitotic agents and rapidly cause the death of both microbial and mammalian cells. Their medical use is confined to anticancer therapy. The biocidal activity of these compounds depends upon a highly specific interaction with DNA.

Continuous monitoring of the optical absorbance at 260 nm of

Figure 4.12 a Mitomycin C (R=H) and porfiromycin (R=CH$_3$). Enzymically generated hydroquinones b are thought to be converted to the reactive quinone methides c which are then subject to nucleophilic attack by purine bases at the indicated positions.

solutions of normal double-stranded DNA during heating reveals an abrupt increase of absorbance as the hydrogen bonds linking the complementary base-pairs of the two strands are ruptured. Once separated, the complementary polynucleotide chains lose their correct alignment in relation to each other. Recovery of the native double-helical structure only occurs when the cooling process is carried out very slowly (this is true for bacterial and viral DNA; renaturation is rarely observed with mammalian DNA). If the cooling process is rapid, complete renaturation is prevented, since correct alignment of the complementary base-pairs cannot occur. DNA isolated from bacteria treated with mitomycin-like compounds shows a very different pattern of behaviour. The absorbance profile is essentially normal as the temperature is raised. Even during rapid cooling, however, extensive renaturation of the DNA is observed.

This property of DNA from mitomycin-treated cells is apparently due to the existence of heat-stable, covalent cross-links between the complementary strands. Although the hydrogen bonds are ruptured as the DNA is heated, the cross-links remain intact and hold the two strands in register. On cooling, therefore, hydrogen-bonding between correct base-pairs is facilitated and the double helix readily re-forms (Fig. 4.13). Addition of mitomycin to solutions of DNA *in vitro* does not lead to the formation of cross-links. Clearly some sort of metabolic activation of the drug is required. Recent evidence indicates that there is an initial NADPH-dependent, enzymic reduction of mitomycin to the corresponding hydroquinone followed by several reactions that lead to the formation of the reactive quinone methide shown in Fig. 4.12. The quinone methide is then subjected to nucleophilic attack at two positions by certain purine bases, most likely guanine, and the complementary strands of DNA thus cross-linking the double helix. Final proof of the proposed interactions with guanine is lacking as it has been impossible to isolate a mitomycin-guanine product from degraded DNA. A preliminary step to the covalent interaction with DNA may be intercalation of the ring system into the double helix. This could account for the highly specific nature of the complex formed with DNA. Mitomycin-induced cross-links in DNA molecules are relatively rare, not exceeding 1 per 1000 nucleotide pairs. Some mitomycin molecules must also alkylate one or other of the DNA chains without forming a cross-link, as there is good evidence that there is about ten times more mitomycin bound to DNA than can be accounted for by the number of cross-links.

Most of the biochemical effects of the mitomycins on cells can be explained by their characteristic interaction with DNA. DNA synthesis stops whenever the replicating fork reaches a mitomycin cross-link. The degradation of DNA that eventually follows the treatment of cells with mitomycins is due to the excision of the cross-linked zones and to the appearance of nucleases associated with lysogenic phages induced by mitomycins. The synthesis of RNA and protein ceases some considerable time after the inhibition of DNA synthesis by the mitomycins. Presumably the transcription of DNA progressively fails as the alkylated DNA is degraded.

C. Drugs that inhibit nucleic acid polmerases

Inhibitors of RNA polymerase: rifamycins, streptovaricins and streptolydigin

All the inhibitors we have considered so far which act at the polymerization level associate in some way with the DNA. As might be

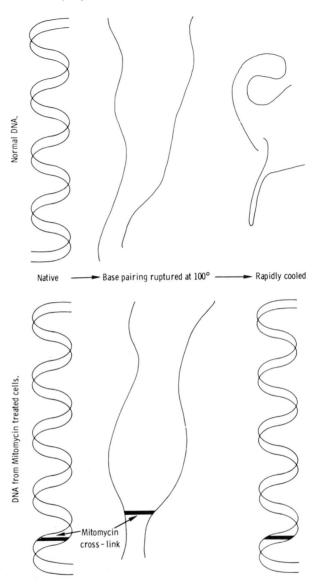

Figure 4.13 Heat denaturation of solutions of DNA isolated from normal bacteria is not reversible on rapid cooling, as correct alignment of complementary base-pairs of the separated strands cannot occur under these conditions. The covalent cross-link in DNA from mitomycin-treated bacteria, however, holds the strands together during heating and greatly facilitates correct base-pairing and hence extensive renaturation on rapid cooling.

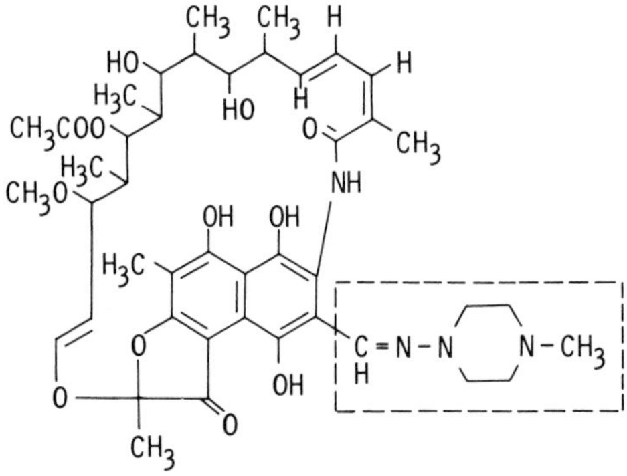

Rifampicin

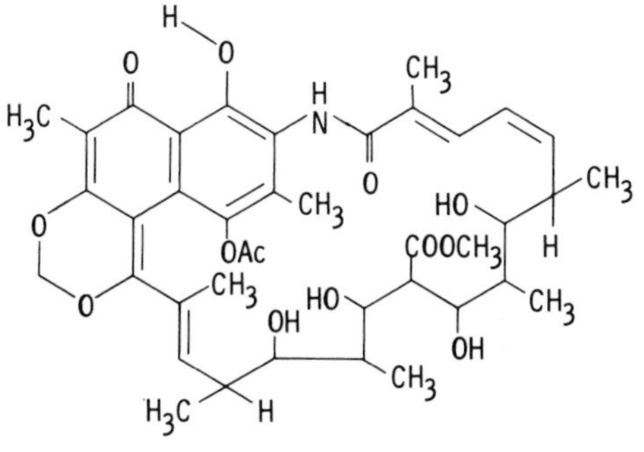

Streptovaricin D

Figure 4.14 Two antibiotics that selectively inhibit bacterial DNA-dependent RNA polymerase. Rifampicin is a semi-synthetic member of the rifamycin group; the synthetic side chain is enclosed by the dotted line. Streptovaricin D is related in structure to the rifamycins; jointly the rifamycins and streptovaricins are known as ansamycins.

expected, few of these agents show useful selectivity between mammalian and microbial cells. However, a number of antimicrobial drugs inhibit bacterial nucleic acid polymerases while having no effect on the corresponding mammalian enzymes.

The rifamycins (Fig. 4.14), first discovered in Italy, comprise a group of closely related antibiotics produced by *Streptomyces mediterranei.*

They have good activity against Gram-positive bacteria and *Myco- bacterium tuberculosis* but are much less active against Gram-negative organisms, apparently because of the low permeability of these organisms to the rifamycins. Chemically the rifamycins are closely related to the streptovaricins (Fig. 4.14) and the two groups of antibiotics appear to have an identical mode of action. They strongly inhibit RNA synthesis in sensitive bacteria and also in cell-free extracts. They do not interact with DNA, and there is good evidence that rifampicin binds to and inhibits DNA-dependent RNA polymerase from sensitive cells. The drug neither binds to nor inhibits the corresponding mammalian enzyme. Bacterial mutants have been isolated which are highly resistant to rifampicin and the RNA polymerase from these cells is resistant to the antibiotic and shows little affinity for it.

Much of the interest in the mode of action of the rifamycins and related antibiotics stems from discoveries about the nature of bacterial DNA-dependent RNA polymerase. This enzyme consists of two major components, one called the minimal or core enzyme and the other the sigma factor. The sigma factor is essential to the normal initiation of RNA synthesis *in vivo*, although it can be dispensed with *in vitro* when certain templates such as mammalian DNA are used. The efficiency of RNA synthesis in the absence of sigma factor is usually much reduced. When DNA from the T4 bacteriophage is used as a template, there is an absolute requirement for sigma factor for initiation *in vitro*. The sigma factor may be involved in the recognition of specific initiation sites on a selected strand of the DNA, enabling the RNA polymerase to attach itself to the template. Rifampicin interferes with the initiation of RNA synthesis, although the antibiotic does not prevent the binding of the intact polymerase to the DNA template.

Despite its key role in initiation, the sigma factor is not the target for rifampicin action, since studies with rifampicin-sensitive and -resistant polymerases indicate that rifampicin resistance is associated with the core enzyme. The core enzyme has been resolved into α, β, β_1 and ω subunits and rifampicin forms a tight, one-to-one complex with the β subunit. The ability to form such a complex is missing in the β subunit isolated from a rifampicin-resistant polymerase. Although the drug is strongly bound to the β subunit, the bonding is not covalent and there may be hydrophobic interactions between the fused aromatic ring system of rifampicin and aromatic amino acids of the enzyme. Recent evidence suggests that the binding of rifampicin to the enzyme is a two-stage process:

$$R + E \rightleftharpoons RE \rightleftharpoons RE^*$$

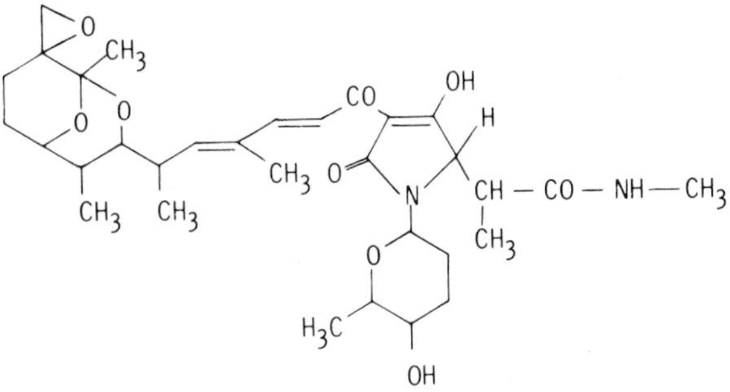

Figure 4.15 Streptolydigin; another selective inhibitor of bacterial DNA-dependent RNA polymerases whose mode of action differs from that of the rifamycins and streptovaricins.

The first stage is a fast bimolecular reaction followed by a second, slower unimolecular process involving a conformational change in the enzyme that is necessary for the inhibitory action of rifampicin. The overall dissociation constant for the interaction is very low: 3nM. Rifampicin has little effect on the formation of the first phosphate diester bond in the polymerization process, but its inhibition of the synthesis of the next bond is virtually total and the drug probably interferes with the binding of an incoming purine nucleoside tri-phosphate to the active site of the enzyme. However, once the initiation of RNA chain synthesis progresses beyond the second or third phosphate diester bond further chain elongation is insensitive to the action of rifampicin.

Streptolydigin (Fig. 4.15), like the rifamycins and streptovaricins, is a specific inhibitor of bacterial RNA polymerase. However, it inhibits chain elongation as well as the initiation process. Streptolydigin increases the stability of the purified RNA polymerase-DNA template complex while rifampicin prevents the stabilization induced by streptolydigin.

The β subunit of the polymerase core enzyme bears the streptolydigin-binding site and the increased stability of the enzyme-template-antibiotic complex presumably delays the progress of the enzyme along the template. The rate of formation of the RNA chain becomes insignificant at high concentrations of streptolydigin. Despite this evidence obtained *in vitro* for the mode of action of streptolydigin, recent studies on its effects on intact *E.coli* cells indicate that streptolydigin *in vivo* may accelerate the termination of RNA chains. The rate of elongation of RNA chains is unaffected but streptolydigin may destabilize the transcription complex *in vivo*, thus permitting premature attachment of termination factors. Only more research will resolve this apparent conflict between studies *in vitro* and *in vivo* on the mode of action of streptolydigin.

Inhibitors of DNA polymerase

Hydroxyphenylazopyrimidines   Although   these   compounds (Fig. 4.16) were synthesized as potential antibacterial agents, they have not found a clinical application because their range of activity is too limited. However, their extraordinary specificity of action against DNA synthesis in Gram-positive bacteria has generated considerable interest among molecular biologists. The antibacterial action of these compounds depends on their ability to inhibit DNA synthesis in sensitive cells. DNA synthesis in Gram-negative organisms is unaffected. The inhibitory action on DNA synthesis has been analyzed in detail and has the following features: (i) Hydroxy-phenylazopyrimidines must first be reduced to the corresponding hydrazines (Fig. 4.17) before they exert their inhibitory effect. This reduction occurs metabolically in bacterial cells. (ii) Of three DNA polymerases that can be isolated from *Bacillus subtilis*, only polymerase III is inhibited by reduced hydroxyphenylazopyrimidines. This enzyme effects the semi-conservative replication of DNA, while polymerase I is concerned solely with repair. A mutant of *B. subtilis* resistant to hydroxyphenylazopyrimidines contains DNA polymerase III which is also resistant to these drugs. *E.coli*, which is intrinsically resistant to the hydroxyphenylazopyrimidines, contains three DNA

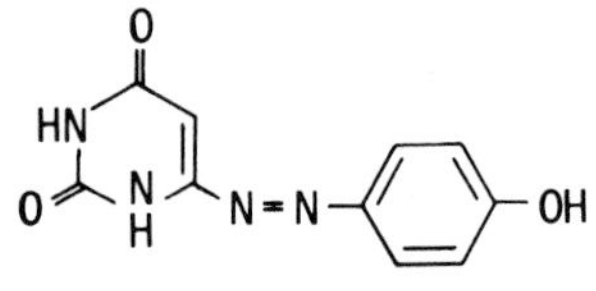

6 - (*p*-Hydroxyphenylazo) uracil

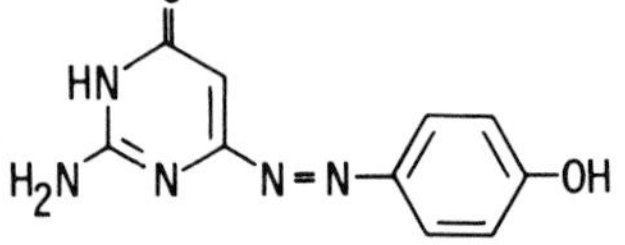

6 - (*p*-Hydroxyphenylazo) isocytosine

Figure 4.16 Two related synthetic chemicals that selectivity inhibit DNA polymerase III of Gram-positive bacteria.

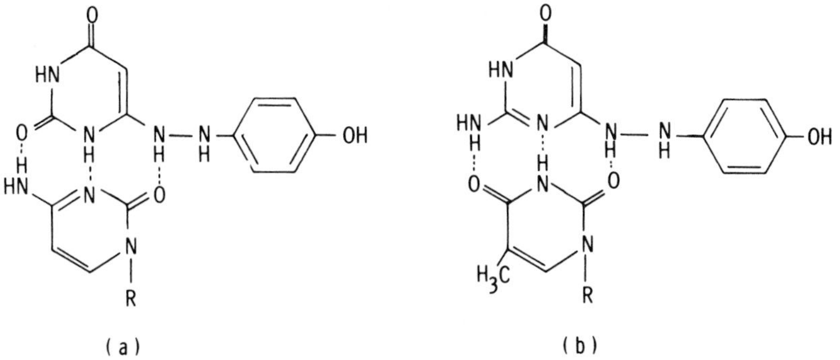

Figure 4.17 A possible mechanism of base-pairing between arylhydrazino-pyrimidines and pyrimidines of the DNA template; a cytosine:hydroxyphenyl-hydrazinouracil, b thymine:hydroxyphenylhydrazinoisocytosine. R is the remainder of nucleotide residue. By interacting simultaneously with DNA polymerase and pyrimidine residues in the DNA template, it is believed that the arylhydrazinopyrimidines prevent purine substrates from binding to the active triphosphate sites.

polymerases that correspond to those from *B. subtilis*. None of these *E.coli* enzymes is inhibited by the pyrimidine derivatives. (iii) The inhibition of *B. subtilis* DNA polymerase III by reduced 6-(*p*-hydroxyphenylazo)uracil (HPUra) is competitively and specifically antagonized by dGTP, while the inhibition by reduced 6-(*p*-hydroxy-phenylazo)isocytosine (HPIso) is relieved by dATP but not by dGTP. These results, together with a study of the n.m.r. spectra of the reduced hydroxyphenylazopyrimidines in the presence and absence of various purine and pyrimidine bases, nucleosides and nucleotides, suggest that the inhibitors interact with both the poly-merase and the DNA template. The interaction with DNA depends on the unusual base-pairing arrangement illustrated in Fig. 4.17 in which HPUra pairs with cytosine and HPIso with thymine. This base-pairing would prevent the access of purine deoxynucleoside triphosphate substrates to their appropriate sites on the template. The ability of dGTP and of dATP to antagonize respectively HPUra and HPIso is the thus neatly accounted for. Complex formation between the drugs and DNA has an absolute requirement for double-stranded DNA with a base-paired 3'-OH primer strand terminus and a distal, unpaired pyrimidine in the template strand with which the drugs can base-pair. The 3'-OH terminus of the primer strand apparently gives the complex considerable stability. The aromatic moiety of a hydroxyphenylazopyrimidine is thought to participate in a stacking interaction with an aromatic amino acid of DNA polymerase III in a hydrophobic site close to the active site.

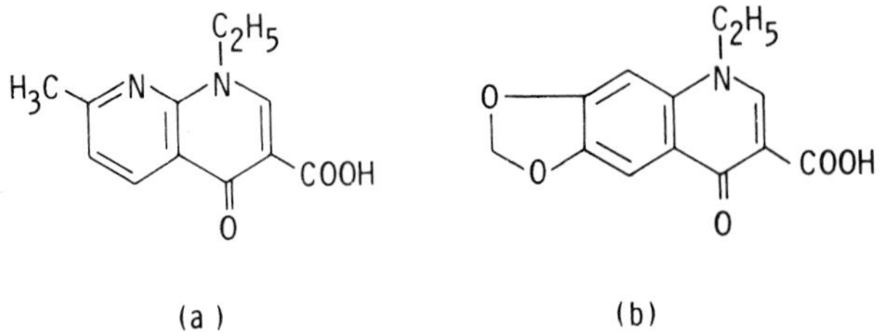

Figure 4.18 Synthetic antibacterial drugs that inhibit DNA gyrase/swivelase: a nalidixic acid, b oxolinic acid.

The unique sensitivity of DNA polymerase III of *B. subtilis* (and presumably of other sensitive Gram-positive bacteria) remains an intriguing problem. The hydroxyphenylazopyrimidines have nevertheless proved valuable in highlighting previously unsuspected differences in DNA synthesis among bacterial genera.

Nalidixic acid   Nalidixic acid is a relatively simple synthetic antibacterial compound (Fig. 4.18) which, has an important place in the treatment of Gram-negative bacterial infections of the urinary tract. Its therapeutic action and that of the related drug, oxolinic acid (Fig. 4.18) depends on selective inhibition of DNA synthesis in the infecting bacteria. The biochemical mechanism of action of nalidixic acid proved difficult to define, but new information about the enzymology of DNA synthesis now permits a reasonable explanation.

The DNA of the bacterial chromosome is compacted about 8000-fold compared with the fully extended macromolecule in the 'B' form. DNA replication and recombination require that the DNA strands separate and unwind the double helix. The astonishing contortions that DNA must undertake in its highly compacted form are initiated and controlled by a number of specific proteins, and the reader is referred to more specialized literature for a full description of these remarkable proteins and their role in replication. One of these proteins, DNA gyrase, is the target for nalidixic acid. We have seen that closed circular DNA can twist upon itself to form superhelical turns. However, superhelical turns also occur in 'nicked' circular DNA and in limited domains of linear DNA as a result of the interaction of the DNA with certain proteins or structural elements in the cell. Two groups of enzymes cause opposite effects on superhelical turns:

(1) DNA 'swivelases' which relax negative turns. These enzymes, which occur both in pro- and eukaryotes, relax the turns by introducing a break in one of the DNA strands, thus allowing the

superhelix to unswivel at the break followed by resealing of the relaxed DNA. The swivelases are unaffected by nalidixic acid.

(2) DNA gyrase. This enzyme, which has so far only been found in prokaryotic cells, couples the hydrolysis of ATP to the introduction of negative superhelices into DNA. In the absence of ATP the enzyme behaves as a swivelase with the ability to relax both negative and positive superhelices. Both nalidixic and oxolinic acids inhibit the ATP-dependent action of DNA gyrase, and drug-resistant mutant cells have gyrase activity that resists the action of these drugs. However, the *nalA* gene in *E.coli* codes for a nalidixic acid-sensitive swivelase activity associated with DNA gyrase (subunit A). Mutations in the *nalA* gene give rise to cells that are resistant to nalidixic and oxolinic acids and also to DNA gyrase resistant to the action of these drugs in cell-free preparations. These results indicate that the subunit A component of DNA gyrase is the target site for nalidixic and oxolinic acids and that DNA gyrase plays an essential role in DNA replication and cell division *in vivo*. There is some evidence that the interaction of DNA with specific proteins associated with replication, transcription and recombination requires the introduction of negative superhelices into DNA. However, DNA replication is probably more dependent on superhelices than is RNA synthesis.

Novobiocin (Fig. 4.19). This is a naturally occurring antibiotic that also inhibits DNA gyrase. Novobiocin-resistant mutants of *E.coli* exhibit DNA gyrase activity that is also resistant to the antibiotic, suggesting that gyrase is the target of novobiocin in the intact cells. However, in contrast with the action of nalidixic acid, the swivelase component of the DNA gyrase is not inhibited by novobiocin. The second component of the gyrase, subunit B, is in fact the target for novobiocin.

Novobiocin has some clinical application as a reserve antibiotic when other drugs fail to cure an infection.

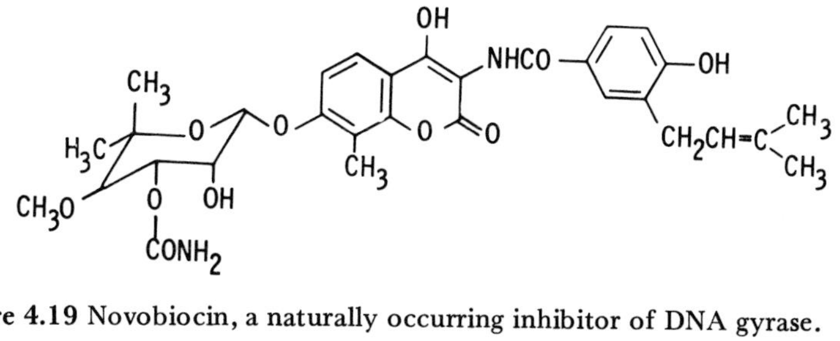

Figure 4.19 Novobiocin, a naturally occurring inhibitor of DNA gyrase.

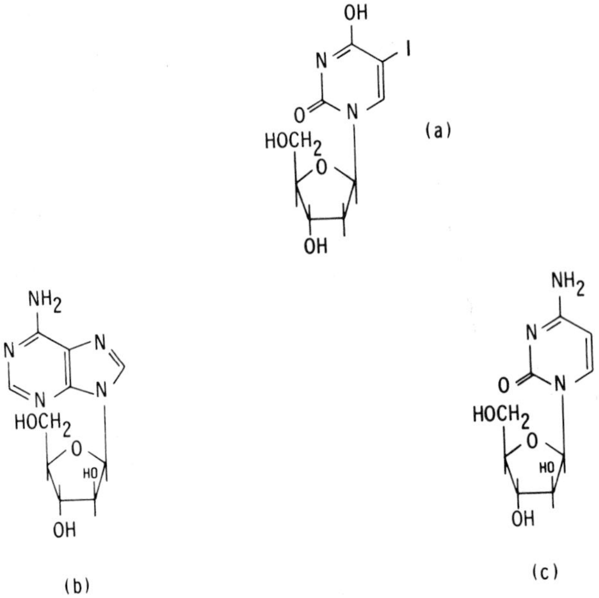

Figure 4.20 Inhibitors of DNA synthesis that become incorporated into DNA: a 5-Iododeoxyuridine (IdUrd), b 9-β-D-arabinosyladenine (AraA), c 1-β-D-arabinosylcytosine (AraC).

Inhibition of nucleic acid synthesis by drugs that become incorporated into the DNA template

Several purine and pyrimidine analogues and their nucleosides inhibit DNA synthesis by becoming incorporated into the DNA structure, thereby disrupting further replication. They have limited antimicrobial specificity because they are also incorporated into the host DNA. However, the compounds (Fig. 4.20) discussed below have clinically useful antiviral activity; two of them also act against malignant tumours.

5-Iododeoxyuridine (IdUrd)

This compound (Fig. 4.20) was synthesized during a search for novel anticancer and antiviral agents among analogues of pyrimidines and pyrimidine nucleosides. Antiviral chemotherapy is generally even less rewarding than anticancer chemotherapy but IdUrd has an important place as a topically applied agent for the treatment of herpes simplex infection of the cornea, a serious condition which may lead to corneal scarring and blindness. IdUrd and the triphosphate to which it is converted *in vivo* inhibit several enzymes concerned with pyrimidine nucleotide biosynthesis and also DNA polymerase. However, the specific antiviral action of IdUrd seems not to depend on enzyme inhibition, but rather on the consequences of the incorporation of IdUrd into the viral DNA in place of thymidine. The similar Van der Waals radii of the iodine atom (0.215 nm) and the methyl group (0.2 nm) enable IdUrd to replace thymidine in DNA with considerable efficiency. It is believed that this replacement leads to base-pairing errors during the replication and transcription of viral DNA with the consequent formation of faulty viral proteins and the eventual termination of the virus infection.

Arabinosylcytosine and arabinosyladenine

1β-D-Arabinosylcytosine (AraC) is a synthetic chemical, whereas 9β-D-arabinosyladenine (AraA) is a natural antibiotic produced by *Streptomyces antibioticus*. Both compounds (Fig. 4.20) have limited clinical usefulness as antivirals (against DNA viruses or viruses with a DNA phase in their lifecycle) and as anticancer agents. Many enzymes are inhibited by AraC and AraA. However, there is little doubt that the biological effects of these compounds depend on their inhibition of DNA synthesis. They must first be converted to the nucleoside triphosphates before inhibition of DNA synthesis can occur. Both analogues are incorporated into DNA and to a limited extent into RNA. The incorporation into DNA and the inhibition of DNA synthesis are competitively antagonized by the corresponding deoxyribonucleoside triphosphates.

Of the three DNA polymerases of mammalian cells, the α-, β- and γ-polymerases, the α-polymerase is the most sensitive to the triphosphates derived from AraA and AraC. It is interesting that DNA polymerase I of *E.coli* is completely insensitive to the analogues while polymerases II and III are partially sensitive. Mutants of *E.coli* and *B.subtilis* deficient in DNA polymerase I are more sensitive to AraA and AraC than are the wild-type organisms. The resistance of the wild-type bacteria is probably due to the ability of DNA polymerase I to repair lesions introduced into the DNA template by the incorporation of AraA or AraC.

How do AraA and AraC inhibit DNA synthesis? Probably two mechanisms are involved: (1) The triphosphate derivatives of AraA and AraC competitively inhibit the incorporation of the corresponding deoxyribonucleoside triphosphates into the DNA chains. (2) The incorporation of the arabinosyl analogues into DNA retards further chain extension at the $3'$-OH terminus of the primer strand. Chain extension does, however, proceed beyond the point of incorporation of the inhibitors as they are frequently found in internucleotide linkages in DNA.

As can be seen in Fig. 4.20, the D-arabinose moiety has an additional hydroxyl group compared with D-deoxyribose. This extra hydroxyl group and a different ring 'pucker' from deoxyribose alter the conformation of the terminal residue of the primer which interacts selectively with the active site of DNA polymerase. Not surprisingly, therefore, the incorporation of the arabinosyl derivatives hinders chain propagation.

Further reading

General

J-i. TOMIZAWA and G. SELZER (1979), 'Initiation of DNA synthesis in *Escherichia coli*', in *Annu. Rev. Biochem.*, **48**, 999.

S.H. WICKNER (1978), 'DNA replication proteins of *Escherichia coli*', in *Annu. Rev. Biochem.*, **47**, 1103.

R. LOSICK and M. CHAMBERLIN (eds) (1976), *RNA Polymerase* (Cold Spring Harbor Laboratory, New York, 1976).

N.G. COZZARELLI (1977), 'The mechanism of action of inhibitors of DNA synthesis', in *Annu. Rev. Biochem.*, **46**, 641.

Intercalation

M.J. WARING (1971), 'Binding of drugs to supercoiled, circular DNA: evidence for and against intercalation', in *Prog. Mol. Subcell. Biol.*, **2**, 216.

S. NEIDLE (1979), 'Molecular basis for action of some DNA binding drugs', in *Prog. Med. Chem.*, **16**, 152.

M.J. WARING (1979), 'Echinomycin, triostin and related antibiotics' p. 173, in *Antibiotics*, Vol. 5, Part 2, ed. F.E. Hahn (Springer Verlag, 1979).

Bleomycin

L.F. POVERK, M. HOGAN and N. DATTAGUPTA (1979), 'Binding of bleomycin to DNA: intercalation of the bisthiazole rings', in *Biochemistry*, **18**, 96.

C.W. HAIDLE and R.S. LLOYD (1979), 'Bleomycin' p. 124, in *Antibiotics*, Vol. 5, Part 2, ed. F.E. Hahn (Springer Verlag, 1979).

N.J. OPPENHEIMER, L.O. RODRIGUEZ and S.M. HECHT (1979), 'Structural studies of 'active complex' of bleomycin', in *Proc. Natl. Acad. Sci. U.S.A.*, **76**, 5616.

Mitomycin

R.W. FRANCK (1979), 'The mitomycin antibiotics', in *Prog. Chem. Org. Nat. Prod.*, **38**, 1.

Rifamycins and Streptolydigin

W. WEHRLI and M. STAEHELIN (1971), 'Actions of the rifamycins', in *Bacterial Rev.*, **35**, 290.

W.R. McCLURE and C.L. CECH (1978), 'On the mechanism of rifampicin inhibition of RNA synthesis', *J. Biol. Chem.*, **253**, 8949.

K. VON MEYENBURG, L.D. NIELSEN, K. JOHNSEN, S. MOLIN, B. SVENNINGSEN and G. MIOZARRI (1978), 'Re-evaluation of mode of action of streptolydigin in *Escherichia coli*: induction of transcription termination *in vivo*', in *Antimicrob. Agents Chemothe*r., 13, 234.

Hydroxyphenylazopyrimidines
N.C. BROWN and G.E. WRIGHT (1977), 'The molecular basis for the inhibitory action of 6-(arylhydrazino)pyrimidines on the replication-specific DNA polymerase III of Gram-positive bacteria', p. 151 in *Drug Action at the Molecular Level*, ed. G.C.K. Roberts (Macmillan, 1977).

Nalidixic acid
J.J. CHAMPOUX (1978), 'Proteins that affect DNA conformation', in *Annu. Rev. Biochem.*, 47, 449.
A.M. PEDRINI (1979), 'Nalidixic acid', p. 154, in *Antibiotics*, Vol. 5, Part 1, ed. F.E. Hahn (Springer Verlag, 1979).

Purine and pyrimidine antagonists
R.T. SUHADOLNIK (1979), 'Naturally occurring nucleoside and nucleotide antibiotics', in *Prog. Nucleic Acid Res. Mol. Biol.*, 22, 193.
C.E. CASS (1979), '9β-D-Arabinofuranosyladenine', p. 85 in *Antibiotics,* Vol. 5, Part 2, ed. F.E. Hahn (Springer Verlag, 1979).
W.H. PRUSOFF, M.S. CHEN, P.H. FISCHER and T.S. LIN (1979), '5-Iodo-2'-deoxyuridine', p. 236, in *Antibiotics*, Vol. 5, Part 2, ed. F.E. Hahn (Springer Verlag, 1979).

5

Suppression of gene function 2. Interference with the translation of the genetic message: Inhibitors of protein synthesis

Many antimicrobial substances inhibit protein biosynthesis. In most instances studied so far, the inhibition involves one or other of the events which take place on the ribosomes. Only a few agents have been described which inhibit either amino acid activation or the attachment of the activated amino acid to the terminal adenylic acid residue of transfer RNA (tRNA). There are many chemical types to be found among the inhibitors of protein synthesis, a fact which has increased the difficulty of understanding the molecular nature of their inhibitory effects. Indeed, while the reaction which is inhibited has been identified with some precision in certain instances, the nature of the molecular interaction between the sensitive site and inhibitor remains generally elusive.

The reason lies in the complexity of the reactions leading to the formation of correctly sequenced polypeptides on the ribosome and also in the complexity of the structure of the ribosome itself. Our intention is to provide an outline of the current knowledge of the steps in protein biosynthesis. More detailed discussion is given to those specific reactions which are blocked by the inhibitors of protein biosynthesis.

Ribosomes

These remarkable organelles are the machines upon which polypeptides are elaborated. There are three main classes of ribosomes identified by their sedimentation coefficients. The 80S ribosomes are apparently confined to eukaryotic cells, while 70S ribosomes are found in both prokaryotic and eukaryotic cells; a unique species of 55S ribosomes found only in mammalian mitochondria resembles bacterial ribosomes in functional organization and antibiotic sensitivity. The 80S particle dissociates reversibly into 60S and 40S subunits and the 70S into 50S and 30S subunits as the Mg^{2+}

concentration of the solution is reduced. Both 80S and 70S ribosomes are composed exclusively of protein and RNA in ratios of approximately 50:50 and 40:60 respectively. There are three distinct species of RNA in most ribosomes, with sedimentation coefficients of 29S, 18S and 5S in 80S particles from animal cells, 25S, 16S and 5S in 80S particles from plant cells and 23S, 16S and 5S in 70S particles; 55S ribosomes contain two RNA species that sediment at about 16S and 12S. In common with the 70S ribosomes of fungal mitochondria, it is doubtful whether 55S ribosomes contain 5S RNA. The protein composition of ribosomes is impressively complex. The 30S subunit of *E.coli* ribosomes contains 21 proteins ('S' proteins), and the 50S subunit 34 proteins ('L' proteins). The amino acid sequences of many of these proteins are already known and work is in progress to determine the sequences of the others. The disposition of all these proteins in the ribosomal subunits is gradually being worked out by a variety of techniques and the reader is referred to more detailed reviews for a full description of this fascinating area of research. Progress with the more complex 80S ribosomes has been slower, as there are between 70 and 80 proteins in these particles. Most of the 80S ribosomal proteins are larger than those of 70S particles, and there is little immunological cross-reactivity between the two sets of proteins, indicating a wide evolutionary divergence. As we shall see, several medically important antibiotics owe their selective antimicrobial action to a specific attack on bacterial 70S ribosomes, while the 80S particles are left unaffected. These differences in ribosomal sensitivities to some antibiotics are almost certainly due to the differences between 70S and 80S proteins. The nature and role of the various types of ribosomal RNA are still uncertain, although it seems likely that 5S RNA interacts with aminoacyl-tRNA and 16S RNA with messenger RNA (mRNA).

Stages in protein biosynthesis

Formation of aminoacyl transfer RNA

Each amino acid is converted by a specific aminoacyl-tRNA synthetase to an aminoacyladenylate which is stabilized by association with the enzyme:

$$ATP + Amino\ acid\ (aa) \xrightleftharpoons{Enzyme} aa-AMP-Enz + PPi$$

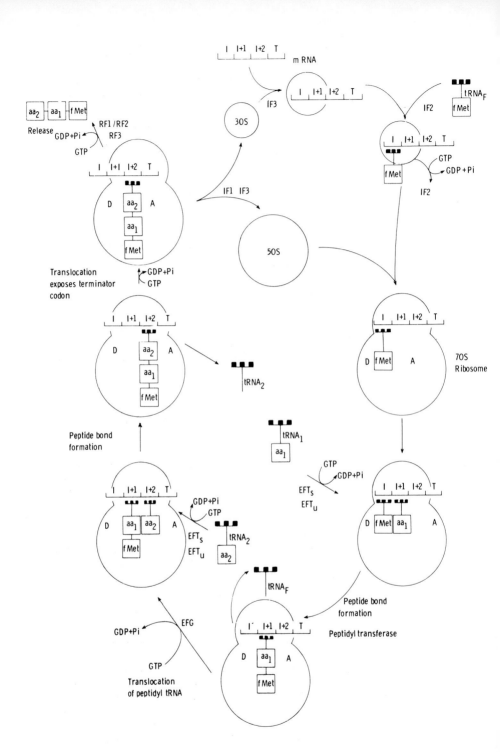

Each amino acid-adenylate-enzyme complex then interacts with an amino acid-specific tRNA to form an aminoacyl-tRNA in which the aminoacyl group is linked to the 3'-OH ribosyl moiety of the 3' terminal adenosyl group of the tRNA by a highly reactive ester bond.

$$\text{aa-AMP-Enz + tRNA} \longrightarrow \text{aminoacyl-tRNA + AMP + Enz}$$

Initiation

The mechanism of initiation has been analysed in detail. Three protein factors, IF1, IF2 and IF3 loosely associated with the 70S ribosome are concerned with initiation. Both IF1 and IF3 have a role in promoting the dissociation of 70S ribosomes, released from previous rounds of polypeptide synthesis, into 30S and 50S subunits. Factor IF3 which then binds to the 30S subunit is also needed for the binding of natural mRNA, although not for the binding of an artificial messenger such as polyU. After this the precise sequence of events is uncertain. The complex containing the 30S subunit, IF3 and mRNA is probably joined by IF2, GTP and the specific initiator tRNA, N-formylmethionyl-tRNA$_F$ (fMet-tRNA$_F$), the role of IF2 being to direct the binding of f Met-tRNA$_F$ to the specific initiator codon, AUG, site. Factor IF1 now promotes the release of IF2 from the complex; if this does not occur, further progression towards peptide bond formation is blocked. The ejection of IF2 requires the hydrolysis of one molecule of GTP to GDP and inorganic phosphate. The next stage probably involves the detachment of IF3 before a 50S subunit joins the complex to form a 70S particle. The association of the 50S and 30S subunits is believed to involve inter-actions between the RNA chains of the respective particles.

Initiation on 80S ribosomes is thought to resemble that on 70S ribosomes except that eukaryotic initiation *in vivo* uses unformylated Met-tRNA^{Met}. In addition, the roles of the specific eukaryotic protein factors, of which there are at least six in initiation on 80S ribosomes, are less clearly defined than in the 70S ribosome system.

Figure 5.1 Diagrammatic scheme of major steps in polypeptide formation on a 70S ribosome. The scheme should be read clockwise starting at the top centre. I, I + 1, I + 2 represent initiator and successive codons and T a terminator codon on mRNA, fMet, aa$_1$ and aa$_2$ represent N-formylmethionine and two other amino acids and tRNA$_F$, tRNA$_1$ and tRNA$_2$ their specific transfer RNAs. A and D are the acceptor and donor sites. The involvement of the various protein cofactors referred to in the text is also indicated.

Peptide bond synthesis and chain elongation

Our present view of polypeptide synthesis rests largely on the concept of two distinct sites on the ribosome which are usually called the acceptor (sometimes aminoacyl or A) site and the donor (sometimes peptidyl or P) site (Fig. 5.1). The acceptor site is the primary decoding site where the codon of the mRNA first interacts with the anticodon region of the specific aminoacyl-tRNA. In the case of fMet-tRNA$_F$, however, binding occurs directly to the donor site. The binding of the next aminoacyl-tRNA to the acceptor site requires protein factors EFT$_s$ and EFT$_u$. The unstable factor, EFT$_u$, binds GTP and then forms a ternary complex with aminoacyl-tRNA. This complex binds to the acceptor site, with accompanying hydrolysis of one molecule of GTP. GTP hydrolysis is not essential for the binding of aminoacyl-tRNA, but in its absence the bound aminoacyl-tRNA is not available for peptide bond formation. The role of the stable factor, EFT$_s$, is to regenerate EFT$_u$-GTP from EFT$_u$-GDP by stimulating the exchange of bound GDP for a molecule of free GTP. Apparently, EFT$_s$ forms a high-affinity intermediate complex with EFT$_s$, and GDP is lost from this intermediate.

The scene is now set for the formation of the first peptide bond. The carboxyl group of the *N*-formyl methionine attached to the donor site through its tRNA is 'donated' to the amino group of the adjacent amino acid at the acceptor site to form a peptide bond. The formation of the peptide bond is catalysed by peptidyl transferase which is a complex component of the 50S subunit, involving proteins L11 and L16. The resultant dipeptide remains attached through its *C*-terminus to the second tRNA at the acceptor site. With the codon-anticodon interaction remaining intact, the dipeptidyl-tRNA is translocated from the acceptor to the donor site as the latter site is vacated by the deacylated tRNA. The third consecutive codon of the mRNA is now exposed at the acceptor site by the relative movement of the ribosome towards the 3' end of the mRNA. The translocation step requires factor EFG and the hydrolysis of a further molecule of GTP. Factor EFG (which binds to a site on the 50S subunit formed from several proteins including L7 and L12, must dissociate from the ribosome between each translocation event. The hydrolysis of GTP, associated with translocation, is essential for the displacement of EFG.

All of the work done so far on peptide bond formation and chain elongation on 80S ribosomes points to a general similarity to 70S ribosomes, although it is certain that there are differences of detail.

Chain termination and release

The signal for termination of the polypeptide chain is given by the appearance of one of three terminator or 'nonsense' codons, UAA, UAG or UGA, at the acceptor site. The complete polypeptide is detached from the tRNA at the C-terminal amino acid, a step that requires peptidyl transferase activity and the release factors RF1, RF2 and RF3. Factors RF1 and RF2 are concerned with the recognition of specific terminator codons, RF1 recognizing UAA and UAG and RF2, UAA and UGA. Both the binding of RF1 and RF2 to the ribosomes and their release require RF3. Cleavage of GTP is also involved in the release reaction. Release from eukaryotic ribosomes involves only one codon-recognizing release factor. There is also a requirement for GTP which is hydrolyzed to GDP and inorganic phosphate during the release process. The formyl groups of the fMet ends of prokaryotic polypeptides are removed by a specific enzyme and in many proteins the methionine residue is also removed. After release of the completed polypeptide, the ribosome is liberated from the mRNA and dissociates into its component 30S and 50S subunits which then enter a pool of subunits available for further rounds of protein synthesis.

Puromycin

The antibiotic puromycin is a unique inhibitor of protein biosynthesis, since the drug itself reacts to form a peptide with the C-terminus of the growing peptide chain on the ribosome, thus prematurely terminating the chain. This remarkable property of puromycin has given the antibiotic an important role in the elucidation of the mechanism of peptide bond formation and also of the mode of action of many other inhibitors of protein biosynthesis. We shall frequently refer to it during the discussion of the modes of action of the other inhibitors.

The structural similarity of puromycin to the terminal aminoacyl adenosine moiety of tRNA was noted many years ago (Fig. 5.2) and this proved to be the key to understanding its actions. Since aminoacyl adenosine is the terminal residue of tRNA in both prokaryotic and eukaryotic organisms, it is not surprisingly that puromycin terminates protein synthesis equally effectively on 70S and 80S ribosomes. The structural analogy of puromycin with aminoacyl adenosine led to the demonstration that the amino group of the antibiotic forms a peptide bond with the acyl group of the terminal aminoacyl adenosine moiety of peptidyl-tRNA attached to

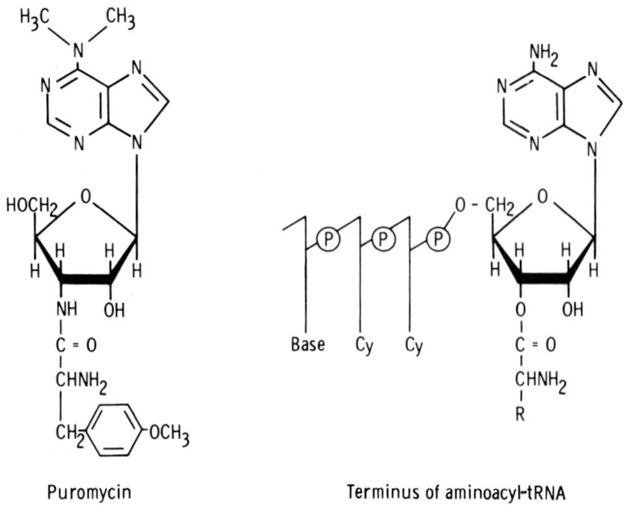

Figure 5.2 Structural analogy between puromycin and the aminoacyl terminus of transfer RNA. Cy represents cytosine and R the rest of the amino acid molecule.

the ribosome. No further peptide bond formation can occur because of the chemical stability of the C-N bond which links the *p*-methoxy-phenylalanine moiety of puromycin to the nucleoside residue. Peptidy puromycin is released from the ribosome.

Provided that the peptidyl-tRNA is in the donor site on the ribosome, its reaction with puromycin (the 'puromycin reaction') proceeds with no other requirement than a normally functioning peptidyl transferase activity. Puromycin does not, however, react with peptidyl-tRNA in the acceptor site; factor EFG and GTP must be added in order to effect translocation of the peptidyl-tRNA to the donor site. Only then is peptidyl puromycin formed and released from the ribosome. The puromycin reaction occurs fairly readily at 0°C, while normal peptide chain elongation is negligible at this temperature, suggesting that puromycin has a considerable competitive advantage over aminoacyl-tRNA in reacting with the peptidyl-tRNA. The reasons for the greater ease of the puromycin reaction compared with normal peptide bond synthesis are uncertain. Conceivably, it could be related to the vastly different molecular sizes of puromycin and aminoacyl-tRNA, since the bulky aminoacyl-tRNA may have to be 'juggled' into a correct alignment at the acceptor site in order for it to react with the peptidyl-tRNA.

A number of analogues and derivatives of puromycin have been prepared and their ability to substitute for puromycin in the puromycin reaction investigated. It is clear that a single benzene ring in the side chain is necessary for activity; replacement of the *p*-methoxyphenylalanine with proline, tryptophan, benzyl histidine or any aliphatic amino acid results in a very marked loss of activity. The L-phenylalanine analogue is about half as active as puromycin, while the D-phenylalanine analogue is completely inactive. Replacing the *p*-methoxyphenylalanine residue with the *S*-benzyl-L-cysteine analogue results in only a minor loss of activity which may be due to the increased distance between the benzene ring and the free $-NH_2$ caused by the additional S and C atoms. Since puromycin substitutes for all aminoacyl-tRNAs equally well, the requirement for a single benzene ring in the amino acid moiety of puromycin and its analogues is puzzling.

The aromatic ring may be involved in a hydrophobic interaction with the terminal adenosine of peptidyl-tRNA at the donor site, thus contributing to the formation of an intimate complex between puromycin and peptidyl-tRNA prior to the formation of a peptide bond. In view of the structure of the aminoacyl adenosine of the tRNA terminus the requirement for linkage of the amino acid moiety to the ribose 3' position of puromycin is, however, not unexpected. Puromycin substituted in the 5' position of the ribose with cytidylic acid is an effective peptide chain terminator, and there is an absolute requirement for cytidine in this derivative. Presumably this substitution extends the structural analogy with tRNA.

Other inhibitors of protein biosynthesis may be classified according to whether or not they inhibit the puromycin reaction. It is, however, necessary to make sure that an apparent inhibition of this reaction is not indirect. For example, inhibition of translocation results in inhibition of the puromycin reaction, since, as discussed above, peptidyl-tRNA in the acceptor position cannot react with puromycin. So far it seems clear that only inhibitors which act on the 50S subunit inhibit the puromycin reaction; inhibitors acting on the 30S subunit have little or no effect.

Inhibitors of aminoacyl-tRNA formation

A number of naturally occurring and synthetic analogues of amino acids are reported to inhibit the formation of the aminoacyl-tRNA complex. Close analogues may become attached to the appropriate tRNA and subsequently become incorporated into abnormal proteins. Included among these are ethionine, norleucine, *N*-ethyl glycine and 3,4-dehydroproline. Other compounds, especially several naturally occurring antibiotics such as borrelidin, furanomycin and indolmycin competitively antagonize the incorporation of the corresponding amino acids, i.e. threonine, isoleucine and tryptophan respectively, into aminoacyl-tRNA. Most of these inhibitors of aminoacyl-tRNA formation lack species specificity and hence have no useful medical application. However, indolmycin is said to be specific for prokaryotic tryptophanyl-tRNA synthetase.

Inhibitors of initiation-complex formation and tRNA-ribosome interaction

Streptomycin

This important antibiotic is a member of the aminoglycoside group and has the complex chemical structure illustrated in Fig. 5.3. While there is considerable variation in the chemical structures of different aminoglycosides, they all possess a cyclohexane ring bearing basic groups in the 1 and 3 positions with oxygen substituents at 4, 5 and 6 and sometimes at 2. All these groups are in equatorial positions.

Streptomycin was discovered by Waksman in the early 1940s and it was the first really effective drug against tuberculosis. Although it is a broad-spectrum antibiotic, active against a wide range of Gram-positive and Gram-negative bacteria, its use has been limited by two major problems. Firstly, bacterial resistance develops readily against this antibiotic; this has been especially troublesome in the treatment of tuberculosis. Streptomycin is, therefore, usually given in combination with two other antitubercular drugs, *p*-aminosalicylic acid and isoniazid, to overcome this problem (Chapter 8). Secondly, when the drug is given by injection (it is not absorbed from the gastrointestinal tract), it is likely to cause irreversible deafness by damaging the 8th cranial nerve. The problem of ototoxicity is common to many of the aminoglycosides and patients must be observed closely for signs of deafness during therapy with these drugs.

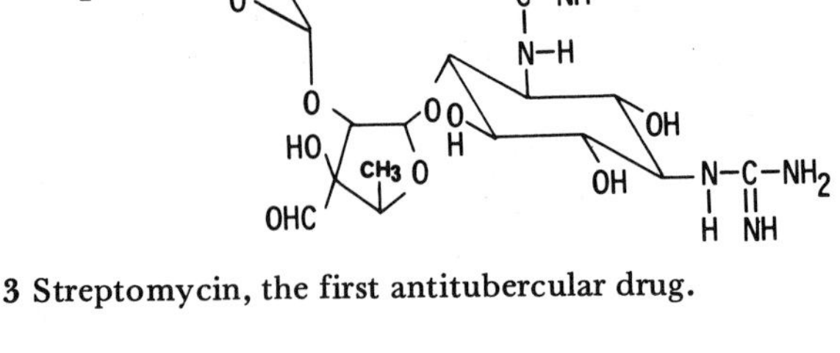

Figure 5.3 Streptomycin, the first antitubercular drug.

Streptomycin is bactericidal, but cell death is preceded by a marked inhibition of protein biosynthesis. The inhibitory effects, studied on isolated 70S ribosomes, are complex and imperfectly understood.

(1) Streptomycin does not inhibit the formation of the initiation complex, but it strongly inhibits the initiation of peptide chains on the complex. The drug also slows the elongation of partly completed chains, but even at high concentrations of streptomycin, chain elongation is not completely suppressed. Peptidyl transferase activity is unaffected. These effects on initiation and elongation are attributed to a distortion of the functions of both acceptor and donor sites by streptomycin.

(2) Many studies have been carried out on the effects of streptomycin in cell-free sytems using synthetic polynucleotides as messengers, and some striking effects are observed. Thus streptomycin inhibits the incorporation into peptide linkages of: (a) phenylalanine directed by poly(U), (b) histidine and threonine directed by poly(AC), (c) arginine and glutamic acid directed by poly(AG). On the other hand, streptomycin may, under some conditions, stimulate the incorporation of amino acids in the presence of synthetic messengers which do not normally code for these amino acids. For example, while streptomycin inhibits the incorporation of phenylalanine in the presence of poly(U), it stimulates the incorporation of isoleucine and serine. Again, streptomycin induces poly(C) to promote the incorporation of threonine and serine instead of proline.

The ability of streptomycin to induce 'misreading' of the genetic code at the ribosome is markedly influenced by the conditions of incubation. The concentration of Mg^{2+} needs to be high, i.e. 20 mM, for misreading to occur, and the concentration of tRNA can affect the level of misreading. Misreading is not random and the following rules are more or less observed:

(i) In any mRNA codon only one base is misread; this is usually a pyrimidine located at the 5′ end or middle position of the codon.
(ii) Misreading of the base at the 3′ end does not occur.
(iii) Misreading of purines is rare and the occurrence of these in a codon decreases the chance of misreading the codon.

Almost certainly, the induction of misreading of the genetic message by streptomycin underlies the ability of this antibiotic to suppress certain bacterial mutations.

(3) Streptomycin also promotes the messenger activity of nucleic acid molecules such as denatured DNA, ribosomal RNA and tRNA, which normally do not act as messengers in ribosomal systems.

Specificity and site of action of streptomycin

The specific antibacterial action of this drug rests on its ability to disrupt protein synthesis on 70S ribosomes whilst having no action on 80S ribosomes. Streptomycin binds tightly, but not irreversibly, to 70S ribosomes. The target site has been identified with some certainty by exploiting a convenient type of bacterial mutant, highly resistant to streptomycin, whose ribosomes are completely resistant to all of the effects of streptomycin. Ribosomes, prepared from streptomycin-sensitive and streptomycin-resistant cells, are dissociated into 30S and 50S subunits by lowering the Mg^{2+} concentration in the medium. A ribosomal subunit 'cross-over' experiment shows that reassociated 70S particles composed of 30S subunits from resistant cells and 50S subunits from sensitive cells are resistant to streptomycin. In the opposite cross, i.e. 30S subunits from sensitive cells and 50S subunits from resistant cells, the resulting 70S ribosomes are streptomycin-sensitive. This suggests that the target site of streptomycin is on the 30S subunit, a view that is strengthened by the finding that steptomycin inhibits aminoacyl-tRNA binding not only to 70S ribosomes but also to isolated 30S subunits from sensitive cells. Using radioactive streptomycin it can be shown that the drug binds specifically to the 30S subunit but not to the 50S subunit of sensitive ribosomes. Streptomycin does not bind to the 30S subunit from resistant cells. The drug does *not* induce misreadings of mRNA translated with resistant ribosomes.

Considerable progress has been made towards identifying the proteins of the 30S subunit of the *E.coli* ribosome that determine the action of streptomycin on the ribosome. Protein S12 appears to be the ultimate target of streptomycin, although it cannot bind the antibiotic by itself. This protein is altered in the streptomycin-resistant 30S subunit. A single amino acid replacement occurs in one of two specific positions in ribosomes from different resistant strains: lysine-42 may be replaced by asparagine, threonine or arginine, while lysine-87 may be replaced only by arginine. Protein S12 may not be essential for protein synthesis, although artifically dissociated ribosomes reconstituted without S12 are markedly defective in translating mRNA which starts with the initiating codon AUG. Poly(U), however, is readily translated by S12-deficient ribosomes. This suggests that S12 is involved in the initiation of protein synthesis from natural messengers.

Although the *target* site for streptomycin action is well-understood, the *binding* site is complex and much less clear. The interaction of streptomycin with the 30S subunit involves at least four other ribosomal proteins S3, S5, S9 and S14. Since a change in the S12 protein alone causes streptomycin-resistance and a concomitant loss of the binding affinity of the 30S subunit for the drug, this protein must also have a role in the binding. In addition, 16S RNA may be involved in the binding process.

Despite the considerable progress towards identifying the site of action of streptomycin on the ribosome, there is still no molecular explanation for the various effects of the antibiotic on protein biosynthesis. Streptomycin may cause conformational changes in sensitive 70S ribosomes which disturb the normal functions of the acceptor and donor sites. Unfortunately, the details of these conformational changes are lacking.

The problem of relating the killing action of streptomycin to its other effects is discussed later in the chapter.

Other aminoglycoside antibiotics

All aminoglycoside antibiotics have effects on protein biosynthesis, although several exert actions different from streptomycin. For example, gentamicin, which is valuable in the treatment of serious urinary tract infections, kanamycin and neomycin (Fig. 5.4), exhibit three, separate, concentration-dependent effects on isolated ribosomes. (1) At concentrations below 2 μg/ml there is strong inhibition of total protein synthesis, but little induction of mRNA misreading. (2) Between 5 and 50 μg/ml, misreading becomes evident, especially of reading through the termination signals. Protein synthesis may therefore increase through the accumulation of abnormally long polypeptides as the ribosomes continue past the end of one message and on to the next. (3) Higher concentrations re-establish inhibition of protein synthesis. These multiphasic effects indicate the existence of at least two binding sites each for gentamicin, kanamycin and neomycin, in contrast with only a single site for streptomycin. Since the binding of dihydrostreptomycin is inhibited by streptomycin but not by gentamicin, kanamycin or neomycin, it is unlikely that the latter antibiotics interact directly with the streptomycin-binding site.

Another indication of more than one site of action for gentamicin comes from the study of ribosomes from a gentamicin-resistant mutant of *E.coli*. This mutation, which affects the L6 protein of the 50S subunit, eliminates the ability of gentamicin to induce misreading of mRNA but leaves the ribosomes *sensitive* to the inhibitory action of gentamicin at low concentrations. It is puzzling, therefore, that the intact cells are resistant to gentamicin. Possibly the alteration in

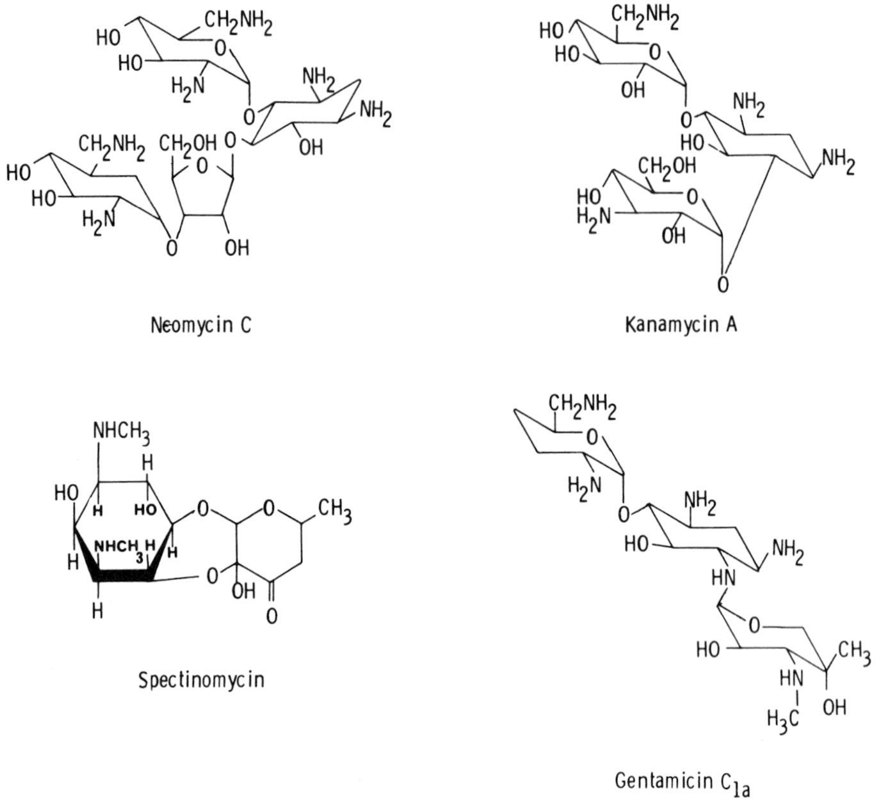

Figure 5.4 Other aminoglycoside antibiotics. Spectinomycin is more appropriately described as an aminocyclitol antibiotic as it contains an inositol ring with two of its OH groups substituted by methylamino groups.

the L6 protein indirectly reduces the uptake of gentamicin into the cells (see Chapter 7).

Spectinomycin is usually included in the aminoglycoside group, even though it lacks an amino sugar residue (Fig. 5.4). Unlike the previously mentioned aminoglycoside antibiotics, it is bacteriostatic rather than bactericidal in action. Its effects on protein synthesis are also markedly different from those of the other aminoglycosides. While it inhibits protein biosynthesis in bacterial cells and in cell-free systems containing 70S ribosomes, spectinomycin does not induce ambiguity in the readout of mRNA. Spectinomycin may inhibit an initial translocation step as it has no effect on codon recognition, peptide bond formation, or chain termination and release.

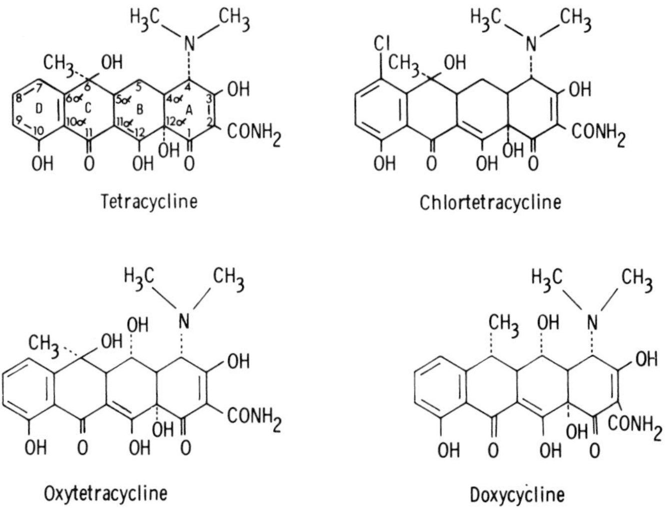

Figure 5.5 Four major tetracycline antibiotics.

Tetracyclines

Four important members of this group are illustrated in Fig. 5.5 The tetracyclines are broad-spectrum antibiotics and, in addition, they are effective against rickettsial organisms and mycoplasmas. The antibiotic activity of the tetracyclines depends on their direct inhibition of protein biosynthesis. Unlike the aminoglycoside antibiotics, the tetracyclines inhibit protein biosynthesis on both 70S and 80S ribosomes, although 70S ribosomes are rather more sensitive. However, the tetracyclines are much more effective against protein synthesis in intact bacteria than against eukaryotic cells because of selective absorption by bacterial cells (Chapter 7).

Studies of the effects of the tetracyclines on the tRNA-ribosome interaction show that they inhibit the binding of aminoacyl-tRNA to the acceptor site on the ribosome but have little effect on binding to the donor site except at high drug concentrations. The binding of fMet-tRNA$_F$ to the ribosome is about one-tenth as sensitive to tetracycline as the binding of other aminoacyl-tRNAs, and this indicates that fMet-tRNA$_F$ binds to the donor site rather than to the acceptor site. The tetracyclines do not directly inhibit formation of the peptide bond or the translocation step except at high concentrations. They have no effect on the hydrolysis of GTP to GDP that is required for functional binding of aminoacyl-tRNA to the acceptor site. Possibly the tetracyclines uncouple the hydrolysis of GTP from the binding reaction. The tetracyclines also inhibit peptide chain termination and release but only at high concentrations and it is doubtful that these effects contribute to their antibacterial action.

Since the interaction between aminoacyl-tRNA and the mRNA codon occurs on the 30S (or 40S) ribosomal subunit, it seems likely that the primary target site for the tetracyclines is on the smaller of the two ribosomal subunits. Tetracycline does in fact inhibit mRNA-directed binding of aminoacyl-tRNA to isolated 30S particles as well as to complete ribosomes. Radioactive tetracycline has been used in attempts to define its locus of action but because the drug binds to most nucleoproteins, it binds to both ribosomal subunits, though the 30S subunit may bind more than the 50S particle. Some studies on the binding of tetracyclines to ribosomal subunits have exploited the property of these drugs to fluoresce strongly in ultraviolet light. This work indicates three strong binding sites on the 30S subunit and a single such site on the 50S subunit. In addition, at least one hundred molecules of tetracycline bind much more weakly to the 70S particle.

To complicate the picture, a recent study asserts that 70S ribosomes have a single high-affinity site which it is claimed may be 'the' site of tetracycline action. The relative contributions of these various binding interactions to the inhibitory mechanism are difficult to assess. Although most of the tetracycline bound to the ribosomes is readily dissociable, a small fraction of tetracycline may bind irreversibly. After treatment with bacteriostatic concentrations of tetracyclines, bacterial cells eventually resume growth when transferred to drug-free medium. Clearly, therefore, even if there is some irreversible binding of tetracycline to the ribosomes, this does not permanently impair their functioning. Because no one has yet obtained ribosomes which are resistant to the tetracyclines, it has not been possible to identify the target site for tetracyclines in the way that was achieved for streptomycin. It may be that a mutation giving tetracycline-resistant ribosomes results in loss of ribosomal function, i.e. a non-viable mutation. The ability of the tetracyclines to inhibit the binding of aminoacyl-tRNA to both 70S and 80S ribosomes suggests that the target site is essentially similar in the two classes of ribosomes.

Once again, the molecular explanation of the inhibitory effects of the tetracycline eludes us. The relationship between chemical structure and antibacterial activity has been worked out in some detail. There is, however, a specific permeation mechanism for the entry of tetracyclines into bacterial cells (see Chapter 7) that has its own structural requirements. It is possible, therefore, that, although

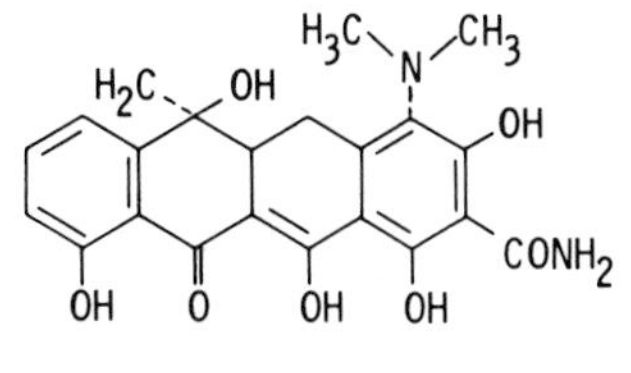

4α 12α -Anhydrotetracycline

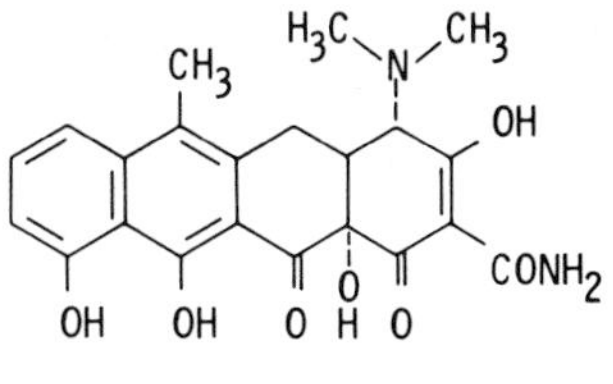

5a, 6-Anhydrotetracycline

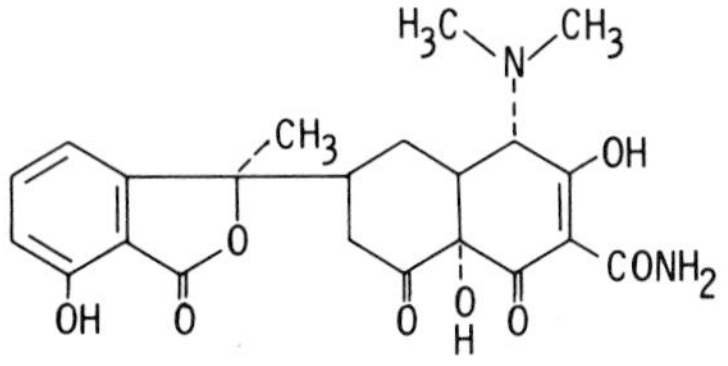

Isotetracycline

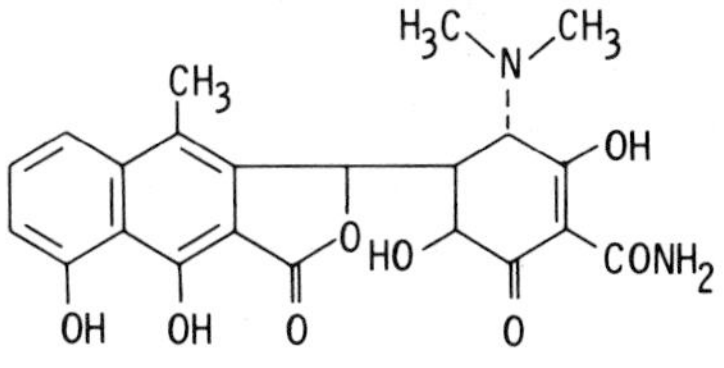

Apo-oxytetracycline

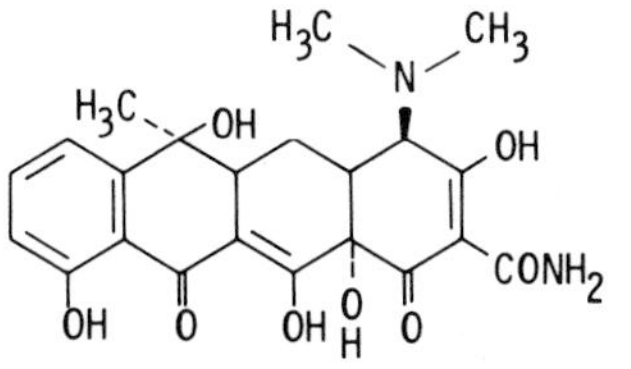

4-Epitetracycline

Figure 5.6 Tetracycline derivatives with greatly reduced antibiotic activity.

some analogues of the tetracyclines may be active inhibitors of protein synthesis, they cannot penetrate into the cell and so lack antibacterial activity.

The limited investigations on the structural requirements of tetracyclines for the inhibition of protein synthesis on isolated ribosomes indicate a number of modifications in structure that significantly affect the degree of inhibition:

(1) Chlorination of the 7 position significantly increases inhibitory activity.

(2) Epimerization of the 4-dimethylamino group significantly decreases activity (Fig. 5.6).

(3) Both 4α,12α-anhydro- and 5α,6-anhydro-tetracyclines (Fig. 5.6) are much less active than tetracycline.

(4) Ring-opening of chlortetracycline and tetracycline to give the iso derivatives (Fig. 5.6) and of oxytetracycline to give α and β isomers of apo-oxytetracycline (Fig. 5.6) results in loss of activity.

(5) Replacement of the amidic function at C_2 with $C \equiv N$ to give tetracycline nitrile results in a marked loss of potency compared with tetracycline.

The ability of the tetracyclines to chelate polyvalent cations may have a bearing on their inhibition of protein biosynthesis. It is tempting to propose that Mg^{2+} attached to the phosphate groups of the ribosomal RNA may act as a link between the ribosome and tetracycline molecules. The concentration of free Mg^{2+} in the vicinity of the ribosomes in the cell will, however, have a major influence on the ability of tetracyclines to interact with ribosomal Mg^{2+}. The 11,12 β-diketone system, the 12α- and the 3-hydroxyl groups have all been implicated as possible complexing sites for polyvalent cations. An alternative suggestion based on circular dichroism studies on chlortetracycline complexes with Ca^{2+} and Mg^{2+} is that chelation requires the bending of ring A back towards ring B and C so that the oxygen atoms at positions 11 and 12 together with those at positions 2 (amide O) and 3 form a co-ordination site into which the metal atom fits. The structural modifications to the tetracycline molecule described above, which affect its ability to inhibit protein synthesis on the ribosomes, may also affect its metal-complexing properties, but no final conclusion as to the nature of the molecular interaction between the tetracyclines and ribosome can be drawn at present.

Inhibitors of peptide bond formation and translocation

Chloramphenicol

This antibiotic (Fig. 5.7) has an antimicrobial spectrum similar to that of the tetracyclines. Perhaps its most important medical use is in the treatment of typhoid fever. However, as described later, certain serious side effects have limited the use of chloramphenicol as a general antibacterial agent. Although originally a natural product, the relative chemical simplicity of chloramphenicol has made its production by chemical synthesis commercially feasible.

The bacteriostatic action of chloramphenicol is due to a specific primary inhibition of protein biosynthesis on 70S ribosomes; it is completely inactive against 80S ribosomes.

Studies with radioactively labelled chloramphenicol show that it binds exclusively to the 50S subunit to a maximum extent of one molecule per subunit. The binding is completely reversible. Structurally unrelated antibiotics such as erythromycin and lincomycin, which also interfere with the function of the 50S

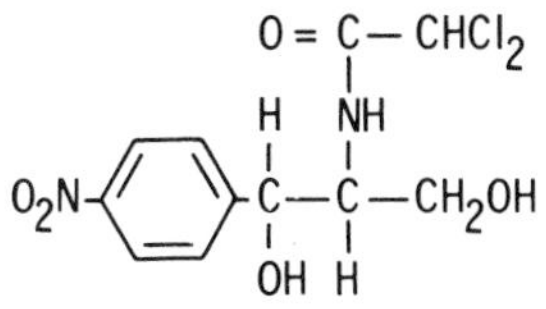

$$O = C - CHCl_2$$

Figure 5.7 Chloramphenicol. The active form is the D-*threo* isomer.

subunit, compete with chloramphenicol for the binding site. The aminoglycosides, which bind exclusively to the 30S subunit, have no effect on the binding of chloramphenicol to the 50S particle. Tetracycline, whose inhibitory action is on the 30S subunit and yet binds to both subunits also fails to affect chloramphenicol binding.

Much effort has gone into identifying the proteins that may be involved in the interaction of chloramphenicol with the 50S particle. The failure to isolate a bacterial mutant with ribosomes resistant to the antibiotic has precluded a direct approach to the identification of the chloramphenicol target site. However, a radiolabelled, chemically reactive analogue of chloramphenicol has been used in an attempt to detect ribosomal proteins that interact with chloramphenicol. This compound, monoiodoamphenicol, in which the reactive ^{14}C-labelled iodacetyl moiety replaces the dichloracetyl group of chloramphenicol, has an action on protein synthesis closely similar to chloramphenicol. At temperatures below $0°C$ monoiodoamphenicol forms a reversible complex with ribosomes that is competitively displaceable by chloramphenicol. At higher temperatures the iodo analogue reacts covalently with several proteins that are considered to form the binding site for chloramphenicol, including S6, L3, L6, L14, L16, L25, L26 and L27. Protein L16, which is concerned in the peptidyl transferase activity and also forms part of the acceptor site, is preferentially labelled by monoiodoamphenicol. Confirmation of the important role of L16 comes from studies with ribosomes specially denuded of proteins L6, L11 and L16. These particles cannot bind chloramphenicol, but binding is partially restored by reconstitution with L16 and binding is further increased by L6 and L11, although L6 and L11 alone do not restore chloramphenicol binding. Some evidence indicates that chloramphenicol binds to more than one ribosomal site which may account for the range of proteins labelled by monoiodoamphenicol. The availability of the two sites to the drug may depend on the condition of the ribosomes during the cycle of protein synthesis. Despite the complex picture presented by the binding studies, the biochemical evidence points strongly to the target of chloramphenicol action being at the acceptor site domain of peptidyl transferase: (1) The antibiotic inhibits the puromycin-dependent release of nascent peptide chains from 70S ribosomes. (2) Its effects on peptide bond formation have been demonstrated with a simplified preparation containing N-formylmethionyl-ACC-AAC (the terminal hexanucleotide fragment of fMet-tRNA$_F$), the 50S subunit and puromycin. In the presence of ethanol (a curious requirement this, and not understood), the dipeptide analogue N-formylmethionyl puromycin is formed and released from the ribosomes; GTP is not required for the reaction. Chloramphenicol prevents the formation of the dipeptide presumably by inhibiting peptidyl transferase.

Chloramphenicol also competively antagonizes both puromycin and aminoacyl-tRNA in the peptide-bond-forming reaction; thus chloramphenicol apparently competes for the same binding site on the ribosome as puromycin and may interfere with the interaction between the last two or three nucleotides at the aminoacyl terminus of tRNA and the ribosome. The present view is that chloramphenicol inhibits peptidyl transferase activity by binding to a complex site on the 50S subunit close to but probably not identical with the site that binds aminoacyl-tRNA in the peptidyl transferase centre. Since the interaction of chloramphenicol with 70S ribosomes is rapidly reversible, bacterial cells previously inhibited by chloramphenicol soon resume protein synthesis and growth when they are transferred to drug-free medium.

Erythromycin

This complex antibiotic (Fig. 5.8) is a member of the macrolide group which is characterized by molecular structures containing large lactone rings linked with amino sugars through glycosidic bonds. Erythromycin is a medium-spectrum antibacterial agent, effective against many Gram-positive bacteria but only against relatively few Gram-negative organisms. The specific antibacterial action of erythromycin depends on its blockade of protein synthesis on 70S ribosomes while having no action on 80S ribosomes. Like chloramphenicol, erythromycin binds exclusively to the 50S subunit. Although there is antagonism between the binding of the two antibiotics, present evidence suggests that they bind to different, but interacting, sites. The 50S subunit can be stripped of both peptidyl transferase activity and the ability to bind erythromycin by extraction with lithium chloride. Of the twelve proteins removed by lithium chloride, only L16 restores both peptidyl transferase and erthromycin-binding activities. However, L16 alone does not bind erythromycin,

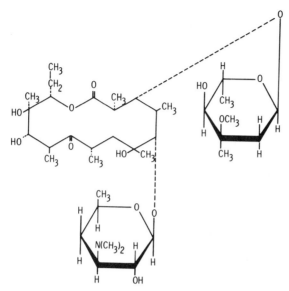

Figure 5.8 Erythromycin, a macrolide antibiotic.

whereas another of the extracted proteins, L15, has some binding ability. In the intact ribosome, L15 may be concerned with erythromycin-binding and peptidyl transferase activity, both functions being modulated in some way by interaction with L16. Lithium chloride-extracted particles probably contain residual L15, whose functions are restored by the addition of L16. Since L16 has an important role in the binding of chloramphenicol, the binding site for this drug and erythromycin must be closely related.

Erythromycin inhibits the puromycin reaction with natural peptidyl-tRNA, but does not block the reaction with peptidyl-tRNA analogues such as N-acetyl phenylalanyl-tRNA and N-acetyl diphenylalanyl-tRNA that have a higher affinity for the peptidyl transferase than natural peptidyl-tRNA. Erythromycin may prevent peptidyl-tRNA gaining proper access to the donor site during translocation while allowing the molecule to bind to a closely adjacent site. Only those peptidyl-tRNA species with a higher than normal affinity for peptidyl transferase can participate in a peptide-bond-forming reaction from this abnormal position. However, this model does not define the precise site of action of erythromycin. The observation that erythromycin inhibits the EFG-dependent ejection of deacylated tRNA from the donor site following peptide bond formation suggests that the failure of peptidyl-tRNA to secure attachment to the donor site in the presence of erythromycin may be a consequence of the persistence of deacylated tRNA at this site. Erythromycin and other macrolides commonly bind to ribosomes or recycling 50S subunits that are devoid of peptidyl-tRNA. Once peptide chain extension has begun, therefore, it is relatively immune from the action of erythromycin.

Lincomycin and clindamycin

Lincomycin and its clinically more useful analogue, clindamycin, (Fig. 5.9) are active against many Gram-positive bacteria but are inactive against Gram-negative species. Although they inhibit protein synthesis on ribosomes from Gram-positive bacteria such as *Bacillus stearothermophilus*, ribosomes from Gram-negative bacteria are generally resistant. This unusual differential sensitivity of ribosomes apparently results from the inability to bind effectively to ribosomes from Gram-negative bacteria. 80S ribosomes from eukaryotic cells are also resistant to lincomycin and clindamycin.

The 50S subunit bears the target site for lincomycin and the antibiotic binds exclusively to this subunit. Lincomycin binding is antagonized by erythromycin, and lincomycin inhibits chloramphenicol binding, suggesting that the binding sites of these three antibiotics are in some way related. Lincomycin apparently binds more effectively to 50S subunits or 70S ribosomes that are free of peptidyl-tRNA. In the living cell the antibiotic probably attacks protein synthesis very early in peptide chain synthesis. The puromycin reaction is blocked by lincomycin, suggesting an action on peptidyl transferase. Lincomycin probably inhibits transpeptidation by interfering with the correct positioning of aminoacyl-tRNA and peptidyl-tRNA at the acceptor and donor sites.

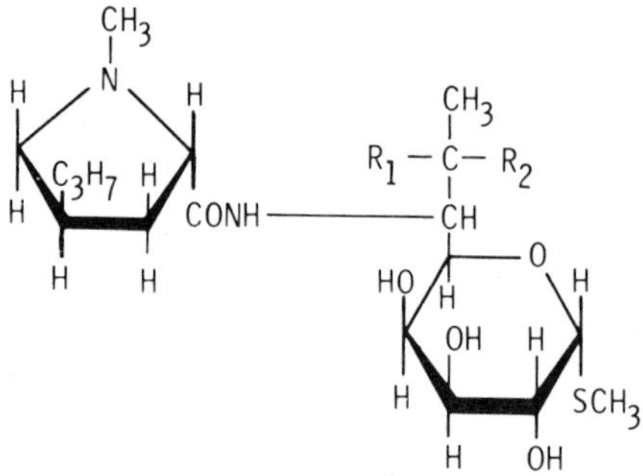

Figure 5.9 Lincomycin (R_1=OH, R_2=H) and clindamycin (R_1=H, R_2=Cl). Clindamycin is chemically manufactured from the natural product lincomycin.

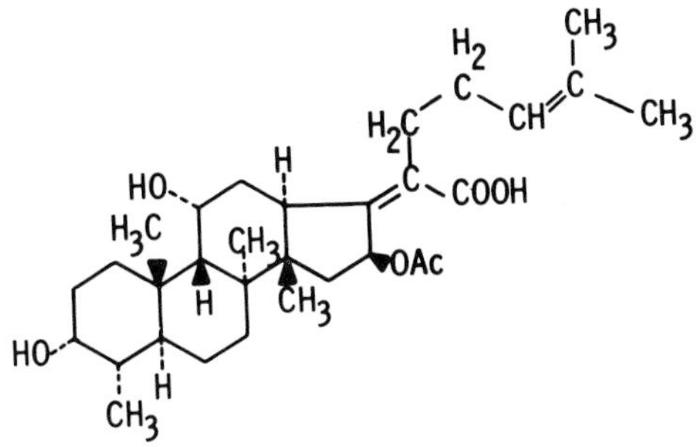

Figure 5.10 Fusidic acid, an antibiotic with a steroid-like structure.

Fusidic acid

Fusidic acid belongs to a group of steroidal antibiotics (Fig. 5.10). It inhibits the growth of Gram-positive but not Gram-negative bacteria and is used clinically to treat Gram-positive infections that are resistant to more widely used agents. Its lack of activity against Gram-negative bacteria may be due to a failure to gain access to their ribosomes since it inhibits protein synthesis in ribosomes from Gram-negative and Gram-positive species *in vitro*. Fusidic acid also blocks protein synthesis in cell-free preparations from yeast and reticulocytes, both of which of course contain 80S ribosomes

Addition of fusidic acid to 70S ribosomes *in vitro* prevents the translocation of peptidyl-tRNA from the acceptor to the donor site and also inhibits the EFG-dependent cleavage of GTP to GDP. The inhibition is overcome by the addition of excess EFG. Bacteria resistant to fusidic acid contain EFG that is also resistant to the drug, and translocation proceeds normally in its presence. All this points to factor EFG as the target protein for fusidic acid. However, contrary to an earlier view, fusidic acid does not directly inhibit GTP hydrolysis. Indeed, in the presence of the drug, an initial burst of GTP hydrolysis can be observed which then slows to zero. Fusidic acid forms a stable complex with EFG, GDP and the ribosome which is unable to release EFG for a further round of translocation and GTP hydrolysis. Work with ribosomes from a mammalian source indicates that fusidic acid works in essentially the same way on 80S ribosomes by stabilizing the EF2-GDP-ribosome complex (EF2 corresponds to the prokaryotic EFG). The lack of toxicity of fusidic acid against mammalian cells is probably because the drug does not achieve an intracellular concentration capable of inhibiting the ribosomes.

Cycloheximide

Sometimes known as actidione, cycloheximide (Fig. 5.11) is unusual, as it specifically inhibits the function of 80S ribosomes but has no action on 70S ribosomes. It is toxic to a wide range of eukaryotic cells including protozoa, yeasts, fungi and mammalian cells. Although this toxicity precludes the clinical use of cycloheximide, it has occasionally been tried as an agricultural fungicide.

Mostly, the antibiotic is used as an experimental tool for the inhibition of protein synthesis in eukaryotic cells.

There are considerable variations in the sensitivity of 80S ribosomes from different species to cycloheximide; for example, ribosomes from *Saccharomyces cerevisiae* are strongly inhibited by cycloheximide, while those from *Saccharomyces fragilis* are resistant. These differences in ribosomal sensitivity have been used to locate the subunit specificity of cycloheximide. Cross-over experiments with the 60S and 40S subunits from *Sac. cerevisiae* and *Sac. fragilis* show that sensitivity to cycloheximide resides in the 60S subunit. Intrinsically resistant ribosomes apparently have modified 60S subunits which are unaffected by the antibiotic.

Cycloheximide interferes with the translocation of peptidyl-tRNA from the acceptor to the donor site on the ribosome and, as with other compounds having this kind of action, the point of attack is on the larger of the two ribosomal subunits. Opinion is divided as to whether the hydrolysis of GTP associated with translocation is inhibited by cycloheximide. The likelihood is that cycloheximide directly inhibits the function of the eukaryotic translocation factor EF2.

Some effects of inhibitors of protein synthesis on living cells

Prokaryotic cells

Most inhibitors of protein biosynthesis inhibit the growth and division of sensitive cells without killing them. Cell growth usually resumes

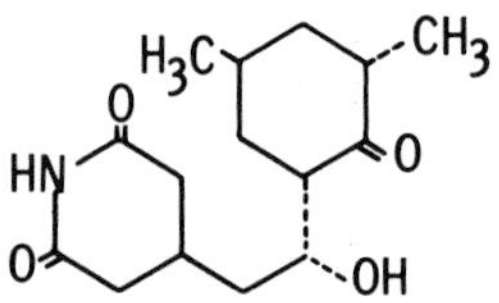

Figure 5.11 Cycloheximide, a specific inhibitor of 80S ribosomes.

some time after the cells are transferred to drug-free medium. Streptomycin and many of the aminoglycosides are exceptional in being excellent bactericides. The basis for the 'killing' action of the aminoglycosides has not been satisfactorily explained. The accumulation of faulty proteins caused by drug-induced misreadings of the genetic code is not implicated because the *ram* mutations, which induce high levels of misreadings, do not cause death, although cell growth is slowed. The addition of puromycin to streptomycin-treated cultures even accelerates killing, even though puromycin itself is not bactericidal and it prevents the accumulation of faulty proteins. The rather tight binding of streptomycin to ribosomes (dissociation constant: 94 nM) ensures that inhibition of protein synthesis is virtually irreversible. The ability of the drug to damage the cytoplasmic membrane and cause the leakage of intracellular ions may also contribute to the lethal action of this antibiotic. However, the cellular resistance to streptomycin of mutants with resistant ribosomes indicates that the ribosome-streptomycin interaction is essential for the killing effect of the drug. Possibly the enhanced influx of streptomycin following the ribosome-linked, drug-induced synthesis of the polyamine-aminoglycoside permease (Chapter 7) in some way aggravates damage to the cytoplasmic membrane, thus contributing to lethality.

Some bacterial mutants show complete dependence on streptomycin and are unable to grow in its absence. In these cells the cationic nature of streptomycin may maintain the structural integrity of an otherwise unstable ribosomal assembly. Alternatively, the mutation to dependence may be associated with a loss of decoding function by the ribosome that can only be restored by streptomycin. In some streptomycin-dependent strains there is a replacement of lysine by glutamic acid at the critically important position 42 of the S12 protein. As this is a change from a positively charged to a negatively charged amino acid, perhaps one of the effects of streptomycin is to mask this negative charge by one of its basic groups. It may be significant that other inducers of codon misreading, such as neamine, paromomycin and dilute ethanol, can support the growth of streptomycin-dependent strains.

Effects of inhibitors of protein synthesis on polysomes

During protein biosynthesis in intact cells mRNA molecules are translated by several ribosomes at once, each ribosome bearing a nascent polypeptide chain. The complex of mRNA-ribosomes-peptidyl-tRNA-aminoacyl-tRNA is known as a polyribosome or polysome. The size and mass of a polysome depends largely on the number of ribosomes attached to the mRNA molecule, and the size distribution of a polysomal population in a cell lysate is readily assessed by sucrose-density-gradient centrifugation. When an inhibitor is added either to growing bacteria or to cell-free systems containing polysomes engaged in protein synthesis, the effects on the polysomal population depend largely on the specific mode of action of the drug. Drugs that inhibit the initiation of protein synthesis usually bring about a rapid loss of polysomes as the ribosomes engaged in translation beyond the initiation stage progressively leave the mRNA at the 3′ end after polypeptide chain termination and release. Inhibitors of polypeptide chain elongation, in contrast, tend to stabilize polysomes as further progression of the ribosomes along the mRNA chain is stopped. Similarly, inhibition of chain termination would be expected to prevent polysomal breakdown, although a specific inhibitor of chain termination has not yet been described. These various effects of inhibitors of protein synthesis on polysomes can to some extent be used as diagnostic aids to identify the site of action of newly discovered inhibitors. Considerable caution must be used in the interpretation of the results, especially when a drug is applied at a concentration less than that necessary to ensure complete inhibition of protein synthesis. When polysomes in intact cells are studied, it should also be remembered that prolonged inhibition of protein synthesis could result in changes in the polysomal population from indirect causes, e.g. increased activity of ribonucleases.

Nucleic acid synthesis during inhibition of protein synthesis

Those inhibitors of protein biosynthesis that do not cause cell death allow the synthesis of RNA and DNA to continue for at least a limited period. In some cases the continued synthesis of nucleic acids provides useful indirect evidence for a selective action of a drug on protein synthesis. For example, the inhibition of protein biosynthesis by the tetracycline antibiotics was formerly regarded as secondary to their interference with energy-yielding reactions in the cell. The demonstration that nucleic acid synthesis persisted after inhibition of protein synthesis by tetracyclines proved that the latter effect could not be due to inhibition of energy production, since nucleic acid synthesis also requires biological energy. The continuation of nucleic acid synthesis also indicates that a drug does not inhibit protein synthesis by interfering with the synthesis of mRNA.

Originally it was thought that the inhibition of protein synthesis had little or no effect on DNA synthesis, since the latter process continues for some considerable time after the addition of inhibitors of protein synthesis. It is now realized, however, that the inhibition of protein synthesis allows only the completion of a previously initiated cycle of replication of the bacterial chromosome. After the completion of this cycle, DNA synthesis ceases. The continued biosynthesis of proteins associated with the initiation of DNA synthesis is essential for a fresh round of DNA replication.

The continued production of RNA during inhibition of protein synthesis by antibiotics is rather surprising because amino acid-requiring mutants of bacteria deprived of their essential amino acids cease both protein and RNA synthesis unless the bacterial strain happens to be of the 'relaxed' variety, in which case RNA synthesis continues. Antibiotics that inhibit protein synthesis in some way uncouple the synthesis of protein from that of RNA. About 25 per cent of the RNA that accumulates during complete inhibition of protein synthesis appears to be tRNA. The major (75 per cent) RNA fraction occurs in particles that contain a little protein and sediment more slowly than 30S ribosomal subunits in the ultracentrifuge. Unlike intact ribosomes and their subunits, the RNA-rich particles that accumulate during the complete inhibition of protein synthesis are very sensitive to ribonuclease and sonic vibrations. While the RNA in these particles is ribosomal in nature, the protein is low-molecular-weight basic material with which the nucleic acid adventitiously associates and is not, therefore, truly ribosomal.

Effects of inhibitors of 70S ribosomes on eukaryotic cells

Subcellular organelles in eukaryotic cells such as mitochondria or chloroplasts in photosynthetic organisms contain ribosomes that more closely resemble 70S than 80S ribosomes both in size and sensitivity to ribosomal inhibitors. Although only a small proportion of the protein of the subcellular organelles is synthesized on the organelle-specific ribosomes, the inhibition of these ribosomes may underlie the action of some antibiotics on eukaryotic cells. For example, yeast cells grown in the presence of chloramphenicol, erythromycin or lincomycin become deficient in various cytochromes through interference with the biogenesis of the mitochondria. Streptomycin and erythromycin cause the loss of the photosynthetic organelles from *Chlamydomonas* and *Euglena* and this may be associated with antibiotic attack on the chloroplast ribosomes. Despite the excellent antibacterial activity of chloramphenicol its clinical use is severely limited by a tendency to damage the bone marrow. A concentration of 25-30 µg of chloramphenicol/ml of blood maintained for 1-2 weeks leads to an accumulation of nucleated erythrocytes in the marrow, indicating an interference with the normal maturation process. Normal erythropoiesis usually resumes after withdrawal of the drug, but very occasionally, i.e. not more than 1 in 20 000 cases, a more serious defect develops in the marrow which leads irreversibly to the loss of both white and red cell precursors. The biochemical basis for the marrow toxicity of chloramphenicol has not been established. However, an action of the drug on mitochondrial ribosomes, with a consequent loss of respiratory function in the marrow cells, cannot be ruled out. The very low incidence of the fatal, irreversible form of chloramphenicol toxicity indicates a special sensitivity in those few individuals who succumb to it.

Further reading

Ribosome structure
R. BRIMACOMBE, G. STÖFFLER and H.G. WITTMANN (1978), 'Ribosome structure', in *Annu. Rev. Biochem.*, 47, 217.

Protein biosynthesis'
M. GRUNBERG-MANAGO and F. GROS (1977), 'Initiation mechanisms of protein biosynthesis', in *Prog. Nucleic Acid Res. Mol. Biol.*, 20, 209.
E. BERMEK (1978), 'Mechanisms in polypeptide elongation on ribosomes', in *Prog. Nucleic Acid Res. Mol. Biol.*, 21, 64.
D.P. NIERLICH (1978), 'Regulation of bacterial growth, RNA and protein synthesis', in *Annu. Rev. Microbiol.*, 32, 393.
C.T. CASKEY (1977), 'Peptide chain termination', in *'Molecular Mechanisms of Protein Biosynthesis'*, ed. H. Weissbach and S. Pestka (Academic Press, 1977).

Inhibitors of aminoacyl-tRNA synthesis
D. VAZQUEZ (1974), 'Inhibitiors of protein synthesis', in *Febs lett.*, 40, 363.

Aminoglycosides
B.J. WALLACE, P.-C. TAI and B.D. DAVIS (1979), 'Streptomycin and related antibiotics', p. 272, in *Antibiotics*, Vol. 5, Part 1, ed. F.E. Hahn (Springer Verlag, 1979).
P.-C. TAI and B.D. DAVIS (1979), 'Triphasic concentration effects of gentamicin on activity and misreading in protein synthesis', in *Biochemistry*, 18, 193.
G. ZIERHUT, W. PIEPERSBERG and A. BÖCK (1979), 'Comparative analysis of effect of aminoglycosides on protein synthesis *in vitro*', in *Eur. J. Biochem.*, 98, 577.

Tetracyclines
A. KAJI and M. RYOJI (1979), 'Tetracycline', p. 304, in *Antibiotics*, Vol. 5, Part 1, ed. F.E. Hahn (Springer Verlag, 1979).
J.R. BROWN and D.S. IRELAND (1978), 'Structural requirements for tetracycline activity', in *Adv. Pharmacol. Chemother.*, 15, 161.

Chloramphenicol
O. PONGS (1977), 'The receptor site for chloramphenicol *in vitro* and *in vivo*', p. 190, in *'Drug Action at the Molecular Level'*, ed. G.C.K. Roberts (Macmillan, 1977).
O. PONGS (1977), 'Chloramphenicol', p. 26, in *Antibiotics*, Vol. 5, Part 1, ed. F.E. Hahn (Springer Verlag, 1979).

Erythromycin
H. TERAOKA and K.H. NIERHAUS (1978), 'Ribosomal erythromycin binding proteins in *Escherichia coli*', in *J. Mol. Biol.*, **126**, 185.

Lincoymcin
F.N. CHANG (1979), 'Lincomycin', p. 127, in *Antibiotics*, Vol. 5, Part 1, ed. F.E. Hahn (Springer Verlag, 1979).

Fusidic acid
W. VON DAEHNE, W.O. GODTFREDSEN and P.R. RASMUSSEN (1979), 'Structure-activity relationships in fusidic acid type antibiotics', in *Adv. Appl. Microbiol.*, **25**, 95.

6 Synthetic antimicrobial agents and compounds with special applications

The sulphonamide antibacterials

The sulphonamides were the first compounds found to suppress bacterial infections. The original indication of this action was shown by the dyestuff Prontosil rubrum (Fig. 6.1). It soon became apparent that activity was associated with the sulphonamide group. Sulphanilamide seemed a likely metabolic breakdown product of Prontosil and was found to possess antibacterial properties. A search quickly followed for more effective derivatives. The first of these to come into general use was sulphapyridine (M & B 693), which in turn was replaced by compounds with less unpleasant side effects. Several of these early sulphonamides are still in regular use, the best known being sulphadiazine and sulphadimidine; sulphafurazole has quite similar biological properties, but has the advantage of higher solubility. Structures of these sulphonamides are shown in Fig. 6.1. Many other sulphonamide antibacterials have been developed since; these are probably no more effective than the earlier compounds, though some are much more persistent in the body and can therefore be dosed less frequently. The sulphonamides act against a wide range of bacteria, but their main success immediately following their discovery was in the treatment of streptococcal infections and pneumococcal pneumonia. They were largely displaced by the antibiotics, partly because the natural products had greater potency and partly through the emergence of bacteria resistant to sulphonamides. However, they have retained a place in treatment, especially for urinary tract infections, and for several forms of meningitis; they are also widely used in veterinary medicine. Later a combination of a sulphonamide with trimethoprim (see below) opened an important new area of use. The structural requirements for antibacterial activity in the sulphonamide series are relatively simple. Starting from sulphanilamide the modifications have been almost entirely variations in substitution on the nitrogen of the sulphonamide group. Substitution on the aromatic amino group

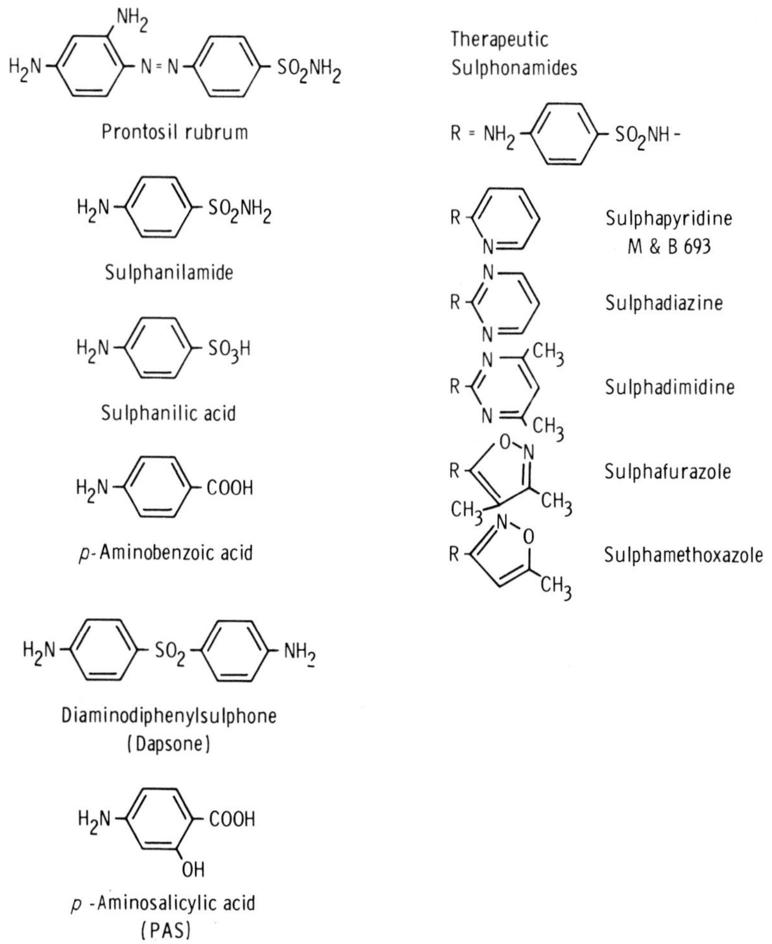

Figure 6.1 The sulphonamide antibacerials and related compounds.

causes loss of activity.

During the search for antibacterials related to the sulphonamides many compounds were prepared and set aside because their activity was not sufficiently high. Among these was 4, 4'-diaminodiphenyl-sulphone (dapsone, Fig. 6.1), which has no useful action against the common bacterial infections, but was later found to have an excellent effect in leprosy. It is still the drug mainly used for the treatment of this disease. Another compound which may be considered along with the sulphonamides is *p*-aminosalicylic acid (PAS) (Fig. 6.1). This substance again is not a general antibacterial agent, but has a specific action against the tubercle bacillus and is one of the trio of drugs used in the standard treatment of tuberculosis. Both dapsone and PAS are thought to act by the same biochemical mechanism as the sulphonamides, but the reason for their specificity in these particular mycobacterial infections is not known.

A few years after the discovery of the antibacterial activity of the sulphonamides some bacteria were shown to have a requirement for *p*-aminobenzoic acid (Fig. 6.1) as a growth factor. When the structures of sulphanilamide and *p*-aminobenzoic acid were compared the correspondence in shape between the two molecules was immediately apparent. The benzene ring with its amino group was present in both and the groups *para* to the amino group had considerable similarities. The two compounds were described as 'isosteres'. A competitive antagonism between *p*-aminobenzoic acid and sulphanilamide or other antibacterial sulphonamides in their effects on the growth of bacteria was demonstrated experimentally and this established the general site of action of these compounds. The exact significance of this observation in bacterial biochemistry was only gradually revealed. The first step came with the establishment of the structure of folic acid, which was shown to contain a *p*-aminobenzyl group. As expected, this unit proved to be derived from *p*-aminobenzoic acid, and moreover the biosynthesis of folic acid could be inhibited by the action of the sulphonamides. The reaction steps were later established in more detail. The biosynthesis proceeds to the dihydropteridine pyrophosphate derivative shown in Fig. 6.2 which then reacts with *p*-aminobenzoic acid with loss of the pyrophosphate group to give dihydropteroic acid. Sulphanilamide and other sulphonamides inhibit the reaction in an apparently competitive manner. The effectiveness of sulphonamides with varying substituents depends mainly on the acidity of the sulphonamide group. The log molar concentration of sulphonamide required to produce a 50 per cent inhibition of dihydropteroate synthetase under fixed conditions shows a linear relationship to pK_a over the range pK_a 5.8 to 9.3. A similar relationship is found between pK_a and antibacterial action, except for the most acidic compounds. Those with pK_a less than 7.0 are relatively less effective, presumably because they are largely ionized at the pH of the experiment and only the un-ionized form can readily penetrate the bacterial membrane. The activity of sulphonamides over the range of pK_a values studied varies about 30-fold. Another example of the barrier to penetration in highly ionized compounds is sulphanilic acid (Fig. 6.1) which strongly inhibits the isolated enzyme but is devoid of antibacterial activity. Although the activity of the typical sulphon-

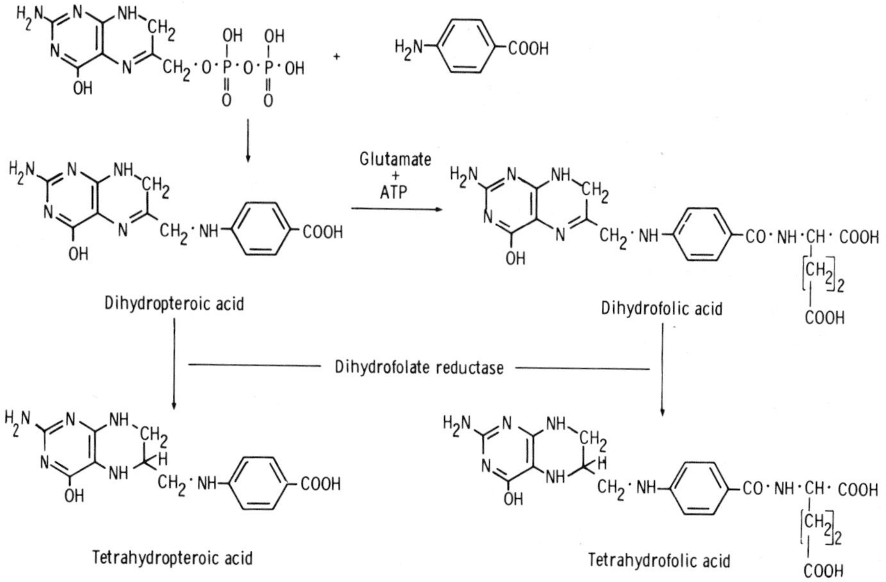

Figure 6.2 The final stages of folic acid biosynthesis.

amides depends strongly on the acidic proton, diaminodiphenyl-sulphone (Fig. 6.1) which lacks acidic properties also inhibits dihydropteroate synthetase competitively and possesses antibacterial activity.

The sulphonamides were originally believed to compete with *p*-aminobenzoate by occupying the active site without taking part in the enzymic action. More recently it has been shown that they compete by acting as alternative substrates. Typical sulphonamides such as sulphathiazole or sulphamethoxazole bind more tightly to dihydropteroate synthetase than does *p*-aminobenzoate. The sulphonamides and *p*-aminobenzoate at equivalent concentrations react with the dihydropteridine pyrophosphate intermediate at similar rates. The sulphonamide reaction products have been identified as the expected analogues of dihydropteroate. Could these play a significant part in the antibacterial action of the sulphonamides by acting as inhibitors of dihydrofolate reductase or of enzymes in the synthetic pathway to dihydropteroate? Probably not. The products do show inhibitory actions especially against dihydropteroate synthetase, but only at high concentrations which could hardly be attained in the cell. Successful application of the sulphonamides depends on maintenance of a relatively high concentration in body tissues. A concentration can then be attained in the infecting bacteria sufficient to complete effectively with the *p*-aminobenzoate available.

The striking success of the sulphonamides coupled with the early knowledge of their point of action led to an extraordinary flurry of chemical activity. Every conceivable bacterial growth factor became the model for the synthesis of analogues that were hoped to repeat the success of the sulphonamides as antibacterial agents. This tremendous effort was almost entirely fruitless. The apparently simple model provided by the antagonism of *p*-aminobenzoic acid by sulphanilamide proved completely misleading. It is worth considering why. The sulphonamides owe their effect to a favourable combination of circumstances that is not easily reproduced in other systems. The natural substrate that they mimic, *p*-aminobenzoic acid, is an intermediate in bacterial biosynthesis that is not normally present in animal cells. Therefore the sulphonamides are not inactivated by excess of the growth factor derived from the host, nor are they particularly toxic as they would be if they antagonized a factor essential to animal metabolism. The end products of the biosynthetic pathway are folic acid and its various derivaties. Most bacteria are not permeable to these compounds so the infecting bacteria are unable to draw on the host's folic acid to supply the deficiency caused by sulphonamides. It was shown quite early that the antibacterial action of sulphonamides was not usually relieved by addition of folic acid to the growth medium. Another fortunate circumstance is that the sulphonamides like *p*-aminobenzoic acid can enter the bacterial cell freely. Many biosynthetic intermediates carry phosphoric acid groups which tend to prevent their passage into bacteria from the medium, and potential inhibitors based on analogous structures share the same difficulty of access. Thus it was a number of properties fortunately coinciding that enabled the sulphonamides to succeed as antibacterial drugs.

Antagonists of dihydrofolate reductase

When the structure of folic acid became known and its relationship to *p*-aminobenzoic acid and the sulphonamides was accepted, a search was naturally made for antagonists among structural analogues of folic acid itself. These were found, but not surprisingly they were highly toxic since folic acid derivatives, in contrast with *p*-aminobenzoic acid, play an important part in the metabolism of animal cells. The toxicity of some of these compounds towards animal cells is actually much greater than towards bacteria since the bacterial membranes are almost completely impermeable to them.

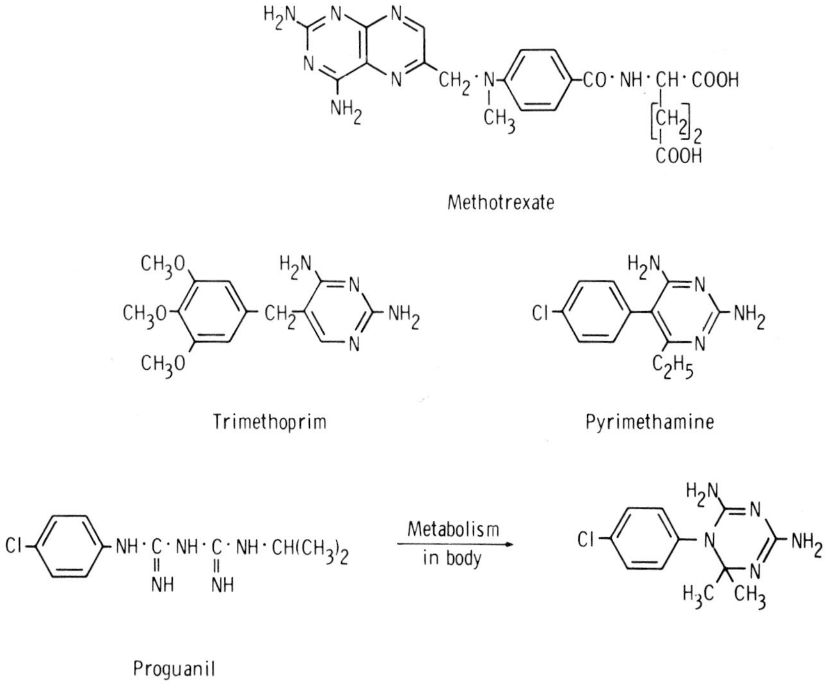

Methotrexate

Trimethoprim

Pyrimethamine

Proguanil

Figure 6.3 Chemotherapeutic agents that antagonize dihydrofolate reductase.

The cytotoxic action of some antifolic compounds, e.g. methotrexate (Fig. 6.3), has found some practical application in the treatment of leukaemia and psoriasis.

Although the direct analogues of folic acid were useless as anti-bacterial agents, other compounds with a similar type of action have considerable antimicrobial importance. This potentiality was first realized in two drugs developed for the treatment of malaria: proguanil and pyrimethamine (Fig. 6.3). Proguanil is apparently not active in its original form but becomes active through metabolic conversion in the body to the dihydrotriazine as shown in the figure. Both this metabolite and pyrimethamine competitively antagonize the utilization of folic acid by *Lactobacillus casei*, and this result directed attention to folic acid biosynthesis as a probable site of action. Antifolic action has been demonstrated in many compounds, their common feature being the presence of 2, 4-diaminopyrimidine or a related ring structure bearing similar substituents; they are clearly analogous to the aminohydroxypyrimidine moiety of the folic acid molecule.

The exact point of attack of these so-called antifolic compounds became apparent when the details of folic acid biosynthesis were fully worked out. The step leading to the production of dihydropteroic acid has already been discussed. At this point glutamic acid may be added to give dihydrofolic acid. However, in either form the dihydro compounds must be reduced to the tetrahydro state by the enzyme dihydrofolate reductase (Fig. 6.2) before they can take part as cofactors in reactions involving single carbon units. Both the cytotoxic analogues of folic acid and the antimalarial compounds mentioned above inhibit dihydrofolate reductase. The antimalarials were not in themselves useful antibacterial agents, but biochemical tests on these and chemically related compounds showed some interesting evidence of enzymic specificity. Although most living cells depend upon dihydrofolate reductase, the enzyme evidently differs in structure from one organism to another, and a useful degree of specificity in the action of antagonists can be achieved. Thus pyrimethamine is not specially active against the reductase from bacteria but has an exceptionally strong affinity for the enzyme from *Plasmodium vinckei*; this may well explain its specific antimalarial action if it is similarly active against other plasmodia. A highly selective action against the enzyme from bacteria was eventually found in the pyrimidine derivative trimethoprim (Fig. 6.3). Reduction of the activity of bacterial dihydrofolate reductase by 50 per cent requires a trimethoprim concentration of 0.01 μM whilst the same inhibition of the reductase from human liver requires 300 μM. The enzymes differ in several other properties; the most striking are summarized below.

| | Dihydrofolate reductase | |
	Mammalian	Bacterial
Substrates	Folate and dihydrofolate	Dihydrofolate only
K_s for dihydrofolate	$<0.05\,\mu$M	$10\,\mu$M
Effect of SH-binding agents	Inhibited	Unaffected

Trimethoprim can be used on its own as an antibacterial but is usually marketed in combination with the sulphonamide sulphamethoxazole as cotrimoxazole ('Septrin'). The combination is claimed to have a wider field of antibacterial activity than the sulphonamides and is used as an alternative to ampicillin. Resistance to the components of the mixture was expected to develop less readily than when either was used alone. This has not been entirely borne out in practice. Both the sulphonamide and trimethoprim block the folic acid biosynthetic pathway, but at different points. This double blockage seems to be specially effective in entirely cutting off the supply of tetrahydrofolate to the bacteria. Deprivation of tetrahydrofolate caused either by sulphonamides, trimethoprim or their combination has widespread effects on the bacterial cell. The lack of C_1 compounds affects protein biosynthesis through deficiency of methionine, glycine and the formyl group of fMet-tRNA and affects nucleic acid synthesis through lack of purines and thymine. The reaction most severely affected is thymine synthesis. When a sulphonamide is added to a culture of *Escherichia coli* growing on a synthetic medium supplemented with amino acids and inosine the cells die through thymine starvation. This 'thymineless death' is preventable by adding thymidine to the culture. The well known bactericidal action of inhibitors of tetrahydrofolate synthesis may well be due to this effect.

Antimicrobial agents affecting terminal respiration

Many antimicrobial agents inhibit the oxygen consumption of micro-organisms. With some compounds the effect is secondary to other actions such as disturbance of membrane function, but with others the action is a primary effect on the enzyme systems that transfer hydrogen from the dehydrogenases to molecular oxygen. The compounds so far discovered that possess this type of action lack selectivity towards micro-organisms; their effect on animal cells means that they are highly toxic and useless as therapeutic agents. However, they have proved to be extremely useful biochemical tools and will therefore be considered in more detail.

Antimycin

This compound (Fig. 6.4) inhibits the growth of yeasts and many fungi but has little effect on bacteria. Cells that are affected by antimycin show an immediate fall in oxygen uptake. Subcellular particles from the rise blast fungus *Piricularia oryzae* containing the cytochrome system also show inhibition of respiratory function. The action on the yeast *Saccharomyces cerevisiae* is particularly instructive. Low concentrations of antimycin inhibit oxygen uptake by the yeast and stimulate fermentation. The organism thus responds as though it were deprived of oxygen. All these results point to an action on the cytochrome pathway and this supposition is fully

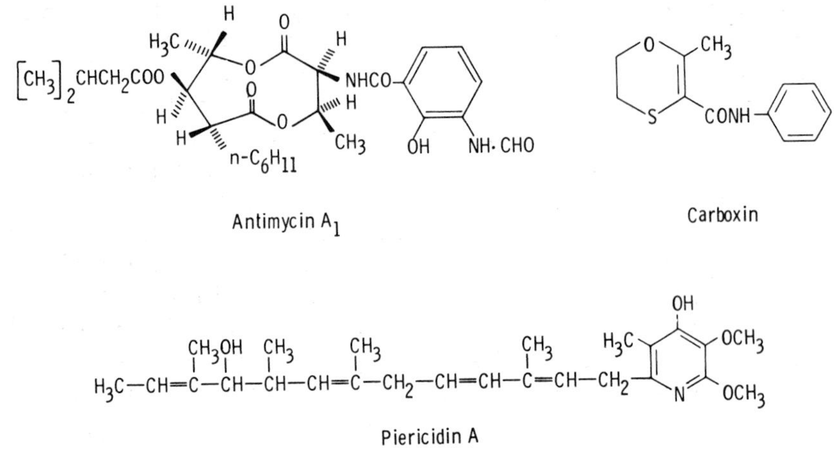

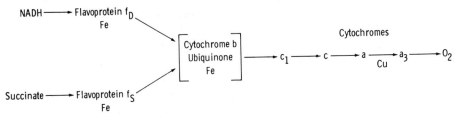

Antimycin A$_1$

Carboxin

Piericidin A

Figure 6.4 Compounds which inhibit terminal respiration.

confirmed by other work on subcellular preparations from animal cells.

The point of action of antimycin has been mainly studied using the well-defined submitochondrial particles which can be obtained from mammalian cells by various disruptive techniques. The sequence of reactions between the dehydrogenases and molecular oxygen is set out in Fig. 6.5; details of reactions represented within the square brackets are still controversial. Antimycin inhibits the respiration of unfractionated particulate oxidase preparations but has no effect on isolated dehydrogenases. The point of attack is further defined by the finding that in these same preparations antimycin inhibits the reduction of cytochrome *c* by NADH but does not inhibit the oxidation of reduced cytochrome *c* by molecular oxygen. The differential spectroscopic method developed by Britton Chance enables the state of oxidation or reduction of all the cytochrome components to be ascertained in a respiratory enzyme preparation. When antimycin is added to a respiring system measurements show

Figure 6.5 Outline of the components of the respiratory chain.

that respiration ceases, leaving cytochromes, a_3, a, c and c_1 in the oxidized form while cytochrome b remains reduced. The block must thus come immediately before cytochrome c_1. This is further confirmed by the demonstration that antimycin inhibits the isolated system ubiquinolcytochrome c oxidoreductase (complex III). The reason for the block is not known in molecular terms though an allosteric type of effect on the mitochondrial enzyme complex has been suggested. The toxicity of antimycin has led to a surprising practical application. It is lethal to fish at concentrations of less that 1 μg/litre and it can be used to clear useless fish from enclosed stretches of water. The relatively small quantity of antibiotic needed for the slaughter is quickly destroyed by light or by biological action and within a day or two a lake can be restocked with commercially valuable fish. This procedure has been used successfully in Canada.

Carboxin and piericidin

Carboxin (Fig. 6.4) is a synthetic fungicide used as a seed dressing to control smut infections in cereal crops. It acts by blocking the succinate branch of the respiratory pathway (Fig. 6.5) at the iron-sulphur protein of the dehydrogenase complex. Piericidin (Fig. 6.4) is a fungicidal and insecticidal antibiotic which specifically blocks a similar region in the other branch of the respiratory chain serving the NAD-dependent dehydrogenases. Piericidin has no commercial application but, like antimycin, is a valuable biochemical tool for studies on the respiratory pathway.

Oligomycin

This antibiotic (Fig. 6.6) and the closely related rutamycin have no significant activity towards bacteria, but are strongly inhibitory to a *limited* number of yeast and fungal species (hence *oligo*mycin). It also acts on cells of animal origin.

Oligomycin reduces the oxygen consumption of intact cells and also of some mitochondrial preparations. However, unlike antimycin its effect is only evident in strongly coupled mitochondria supplied with inorganic phosphate and ADP. If 2,4-dinitrophenol or some other uncoupling agent is added to such preparations, respiration continues even in the presence of oligomycin. The antibiotic has no effect on the oxygen consumption of submitochondrial particles which lack the oxidative phosphorylation mechanism. All these observations indicate that the effect of oligomycin on respiration is indirect, and is due to inhibition of the oxidative phosphorylation

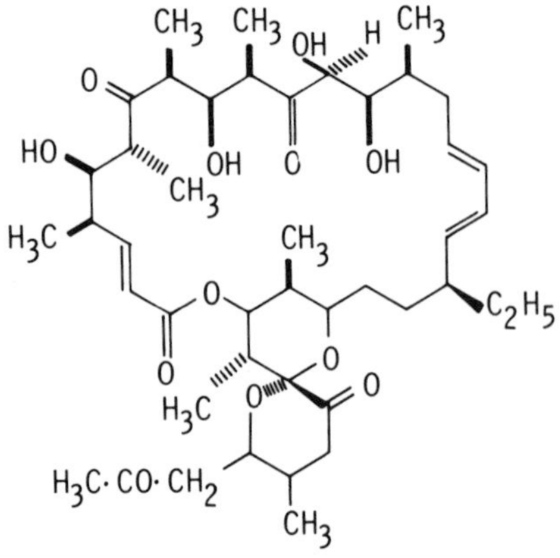

Figure 6.6 Oligomycin.

stages which are normally coupled to respiration in intact cells.

Oxidative phosphorylation is associated with a particular adenosine triphosphatase bound to the mitochondrial membrane. Particulate preparations of this enzyme are strongly inhibited by concentrations of oligomycin (1 μg/ml) which just inhibit fungal growth. They not only catalyse the breakdown of ATP but also the reverse reaction:

$$ADP + P_i + H^+ \rightleftharpoons ATP + H_2O$$

and ATP-P$_i$ exchange. Examination of these membrane preparations by electron microscopy shows spherical particles attached to the membrane by short stalks. These particles can be removed and purified as a protein (F1) which possesses adenosine triphosphatase activity but is insensitive to oligomycin and is no longer capable of ATP synthesis or P$_i$ exchange. The solubilized triphosphatase can be returned to its complete original activity and sensitivity by recombination with suitable inner mitochondrial membrane preparations. One element in this recombination is a basic protein of molecular weight 18 000 known as OSCP (oligomycin-sensitivity-conferring protein). This protein is not the point of attack of oligomycin but is probably concerned with linking the adenosine triphosphatase headpiece to the membrane to produce the complete particle. It may in fact constitute the 'stalk' seen in electron micrographs. The site of oligomycin action apparently lies in the membrane possibly through an association with the phospholipid.

Oxidative phosphorylation involves membrane function and has been explained in terms of Mitchell's chemiosmotic hypothesis. On this theory the effect of oligomycin would depend upon its ability to decrease the proton permeability of the membrane. Such a decrease, by 5 to 10 times, has been shown experimentally in mitochondrial particles from beef heart and in chromophores from *Rhodospirillum*.

Other antibacterial agents

The description up to this point has covered most of the antibacterial agents of therapeutic importance. There remain a few well-known compounds that will be dealt with only briefly because of their mode of action is still in considerable doubt.

Quinoxaline and phenazine *N*-oxides

The di-*N*-oxides of quinoxaline and phenazine provide a series of potent broad-spectrum antibacterial agents, some of which have been isolated from fungi while others are synthetic. None has found a place in human medicine, but carbodox (Fig. 6.7), a synthetic compound, is used for the treatment of swine dysentery and is added to feedstuffs to stimulate growth. These compounds are effective at a lower concentration against facultative bacteria growing anaerobically than when oxygen is present. Under anaerobic conditions the synthesis of DNA is suppressed whilst synthesis of protein and of RNA continue. Reduction of the di-*N*-oxide to a mono-*N*-oxide with the formation of a free radical has been suggested as a possible cause of interference with DNA synthesis, but the mechanism is still obscure.

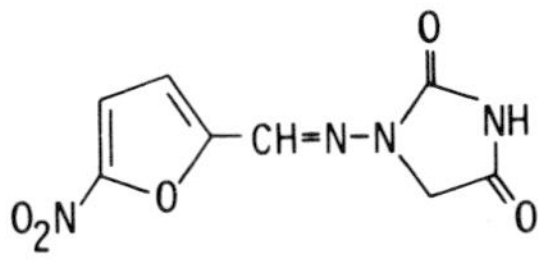

Nitrofurantoin

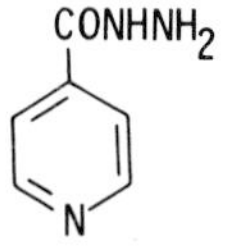

Isonicotinic hydrazide
Isoniazid, INH

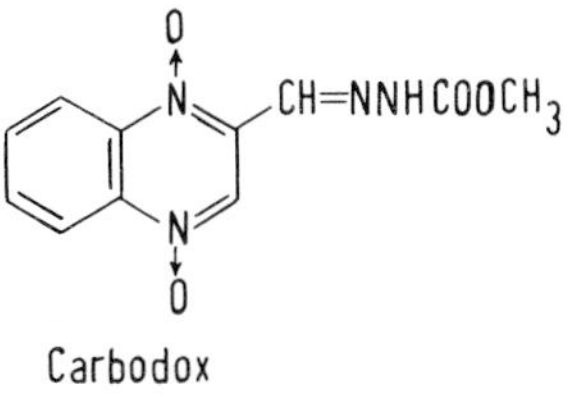

Carbodox

Figure 6.7 Antibacterial agents for which the mode of action is incompletely understood.

The nitrofuran antibacterials

Many synthetic antibacterials based on the 5-nitro-2-furfurylidene structure have been prepared. One of the best known is nitrofurantoin (Fig. 6.7) which finds extensive use against infections of the bladder and urinary tract. The nitrofurans have a wide spectrum of antibacterial activity covering both Gram-positive and Gram-negative organisms. The nitro group is readily reduced by bacteria and reduction may be essential to their antibacterial effect. As evidence of this, mutants of *E.coli* or *S.aureus* with reduced sensitivity to nitrofurans were found to lack nitrofuran reductase I. These mutants retained another reductase which was only functional in the absence of oxygen; under these conditions they were sensitive to nitrofurans. The reduction products of nitrofurans are unstable and have not been identified.

Nitrofurans are mutagenic and cause breaks in DNA. In *E.coli* nitrofurantoin was shown to inhibit the translation of inducible genes, the action being at the initiation step in the formation of mRNA. These seem the most probable causes of antibacterial activity, but convincing proof is lacking. The mutagenic properties of these compounds and toxic side effects prevent their widespread use against human systemic infections, though they have veterinary applications.

Isonicotinic hydrazide (INH)

This synthetic compound (Fig. 6.7) is extremely active against *Mycobacterium tuberculosis* and is probably the most important single drug in the treatment of tuberculosis. When cultures of *M.tuberculosis* are treated with INH there is an early reduction in the NAD content of the cells and an inhibition of the incorporation of labelled precursors into mycolic acid. These changes precede a measurable decline in viability. The effect on mycolic acid synthesis is said to be due to inhibition of C_{24} acid Δ^5 desaturase, a key enzyme in the synthetic pathway. Mycolic acid is a major component in the cell wall of mycobacteria (see Chapter 2), and a block in its synthesis may render the cells non-viable, but this has not been proved.

Sideromycins

The sideromycins constitute a group of powerful and selective antibiotics active against bacterial infections and having little

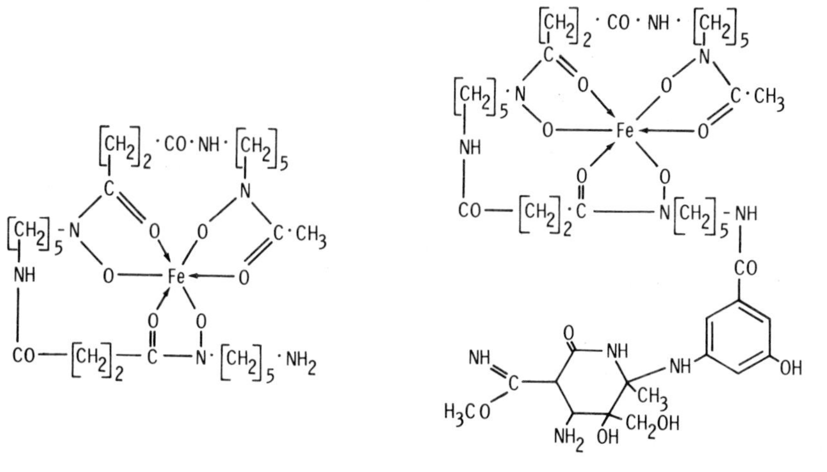

Ferrioxamine B   Ferrimycin A₁

Figure 6.8 Ferrioxamine B, an iron-chelating growth factor, and ferrimycin A₁, a related antibiotic.

mammalian toxicity. They have failed as useful drugs solely because of the extraordinary ease with which bacteria develop resistance to them. They all contain ferric iron in a firmly chelated form and are structurally related to the sideramines. This relationship is exemplified by the sideromycin ferrimycin A₁ which incorporates the complete structure of the sideramine, ferrioxamine B, but possesses in addition a complex pendant group (Fig. 6.8). The significance of this relationship in terms of the cell's transport systems is discussed in Chapter 7. The antibacterial effects of the sideromycins probably depend entirely on the pendant groups, but the biochemical nature of the action is unknown.

Antifungal agents

Almost all organic material is subject to attack or spoilage by fungi, so fungicides are of immense practical importance as preservatives and protective agents. A great many compounds are used for this purpose. The commonest types are based on heavy metals or are relatively labile sulphur compounds such as the dithiocarbamates. These are generally toxic agents with multiple effects, including disturbance of membrane function and interference with respiration. Some of these compounds find use against the many fungal diseases which affect plants, but recent years have seen the development of compounds with subtler effects. In crop-spraying it is a great advantage to use chemicals which are absorbed and translocated within the plant. The antifungal action can then reach parts shielded from the spray and will not be lost through rain. Systemic anti-fungals have more selective effects and a few of the more important have been chosen to illustrate particular modes of action. For a fuller treatment, specialized works should be consulted.

A number of antifungal agents have been described in other parts of this book. These include the polyoxins (Chapter 2), the polyenes (Chapter 3), cycloheximide (Chapter 5), antimycin, carboxin, piericidin and oligomycin (this chapter). Besides these, a number of compounds regarded mainly as antibacterials also possess some antifungal activity.

Fungicides affecting sterol biosynthesis

Triforine (Fig. 6.9) is a systemic fungicide active against plant mildews and rusts. It is one of a diverse group of agricultural fungicides which interfere with the synthesis of sterols. In sensitive organisms treatment with triforine causes loss of ergosterol, an essential component of the fungal wall. From the metabolic precursors which accumulate in treated cells it appears that the synthesis of ergosterol from squalene is blocked at the stage of C-14 demethylation.

Miconazole (Fig. 6.9) is used medically against *Candida albicans*, the organism responsible for thrush. It acts on ergosterol synthesis at the same point as triforine.

Diclobutrazole (Fig. 6.9), an important agricultural fungicide, is yet another compound which interferes with membrane sterol formation. The biosynthetic pathway involves oxidative removal of the 14α-methyl group of 24-methylene dihydrolanosterol through the agency of a cytochrome P_{450}-type enzyme. Diclobutrazole acts by inhibiting enzymes of this type. Miconazole and diclobutrazole have some structural similarities and illustrate how compounds having a particular type of antimicrobial activity can be developed chemically in different ways to suit applications in widely different circumstances.

Griseofulvin and benomyl

Griseofulvin (Fig. 6.9), a naturally occurring antibiotic, is one of the few antifungal agents used medically. It is given by mouth to treat ringworm or fungal infections of the skin or nails. In fungi sensitive to griseofulvin, treatment causes the tips of the hyphae to become

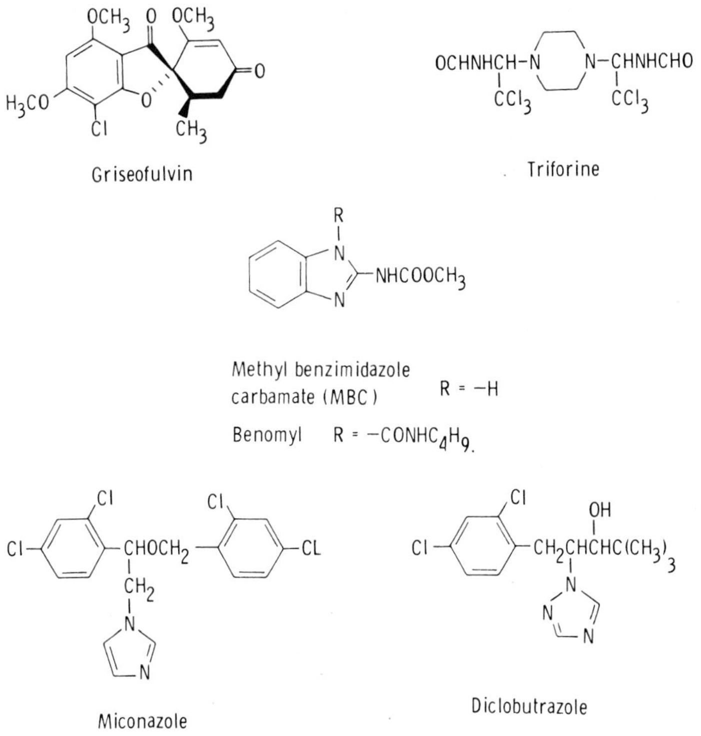

Figure 6.9 Some antifungal compounds.

waved and curled and growth ceases. Further study has shown that griseofulvin binds to proteins involved in the assembly of tubulin into microtubules. The formation of microtubules is inhibited, one important result being the prevention of the separation of chromosomes in mitosis. The selectivity of the action of griseofulvin to fungi is unexplained, since microtubules are common to all cells. It may rest in the specificity of structure of the microtubule-associated proteins.

Benomyl (Fig. 6.9) acts against a wide range of pathogenic fungi affecting plants, and is used extensively in agriculture and horticulture. It acts systemically, being metabolized in plants to MBC (Fig. 6.9) which is regarded as the active agent. Benomyl also affects the separation of the chromosomes in mitosis, but the site of its action is believed to differ from that of griseofulvin.

Compounds used in treating protozoal diseases

Protozoal disease presents a serious problem in man and animals, especially in the hotter areas of the world. Chemotherapy of such diseases has a long history which predates antibacterial therapy by several decades. Many drugs have been developed for use in malaria, trypanosomiasis, amoebiasis and other protozoal diseases, but with few exceptions their mode of action is unproved or obscure. This is largely due to the great technical difficulty of culturing protozoa under controlled experimental conditions, compared with the simplicity of growing bacteria and fungi. Some compounds developed as antibacterials or antifungal agents are effective against protozoa in man. More commonly the antiprotozoal drugs stand on their own and possess little useful antibacterial activity. We shall discuss only those for which a biochemical action can be reasonably adduced, recognizing that it leaves unmentioned a number of drugs of therapeutic importance.

Arsenic and antimony compounds still retain a place in the treatment of protozoal infections. In spite of their long history, the biochemical mechanism of their action remains uncertain. Like arsenite, the trivalent arsenicals react readily with thiol compounds and especially with dithiol compounds such as lipoic acid. Consequently they are inhibitory to enzyme systems which catalyse the oxidative decarboxylation of α-keto acids, in which lipoic acid acts as a cofactor. This, however, is an unselective action and does not explain why certain compounds show preferential toxicity to trypanosomes. Experiments with cells of *Trypanosoma rhodesiense* indicate a marked increase in phosphoenolpyruvate following treatment with 2 μM melarsen (a trypanocidal arsenical). This was attributed to inhibition of phosphokinase, though the isolated enzyme was inhibited only at much higher concentrations. Muscle pyruvate kinase was insensitive to the arsenical. Since the trypanosome relies on glycolysis for its energy production a block in pyruvate kinase would deprive it of its necessary source fo ATP. Similarly, organic antimonials were found to inhibit phosphofructokinase from schistosomes at one-hundredth of the concentration required to inhibit the corresponding mammalian enzyme. Among other trypanocides the action of suramin (Fig. 1.2) is still unknown. This drug possesses considerable structural specificity, and omission of the methyl groups from the two outer benzene rings gives an almost inactive compound. The action of ethidium bromide (Fig. 4.7) on bacteria has been discussed in Chapter 4. Its action on trypanosomes may be similar. It quickly binds to the DNA of the nucleus and the kinetoplast of the flagellated trypanosome-like organism *Crithidia oncopelti*. DNA synthesis is immediately depressed while synthesis of protein and RNA continue unaffected for some time. Once again the reason for the selective effect on the parasite is unexplained since the compound also binds to the host DNA. A possible clue is that blood forms of trypanosomes either carry no net surface charge or have a slight positive charge, while the body's cells are negatively charged. This may enable some compounds to penetrate more easily into the parasite than into the host cell. The antimalarials mepacrine (Fig. 1.2) and chloroquine (Fig. 4.7) which also intercalate with DNA are discussed in Chapter 4 and proguanil and pyrimethamine (Fig. 6.3) have been dealt with in the present chapter.

The modern vogue for rearing chickens in broiler houses has exacerbated many disease problems, coccidiosis being one of the most troublesome. Many compounds have been developed and used for prophylaxis and treatment of this disease. Each in turn has failed or retained only a limited usefulness because of the development of resistance. Sulphonamides and nitrofurans were among the first drugs to be used, and monensin (Fig. 3.7) is currently popular. The action of these compounds on coccidia is presumed to be similar to their action on bacteria. Methyl benzoquate (Fig. 6.10) and the closely similar buquinolate are coccidiostats having structures superficially realted to nalidixic acid (Fig. 4.18) but with a different mode of action. They act upon the respiratory pathway of the coccidia at a point near to cytochrome *b*. The respiration of mitochondria isolated from *Eimeria tenella* using either succinate or malate and pyruvate as substrate was 50 per cent inhibited by 0.01 μM methyl benzoquate or buquinolate whilst mammalian mitochondria were unaffected by much higher concentrations. This would seem to provide a satisfying explanation of the selective toxic action of these compounds on coccidia. Another well-known compound used prophylactically against chick coccidiosis is amprolium (Fig. 6.10). It is clearly related to thiamin and is thought to act at very low concentrations by blocking the access of thiamin to the coccidia in the gut. Higher concentrations prevent the uptake of thiamin by the bird.

Metronidazole (Fig. 6.10) is important in the treatment of amoebic dysentery and trichomoniasis. More recently it has been found particularly useful against obligate anaerobic bacteria. These include bacterioides, fusobacteria, clostridia and anaerobic streptococci. It is used to minimize sepsis after surgery. Its biochemical effects have been studied experimentally in *Trichomonas vaginalis*, using metronidazole labelled with [14]C. The organism readily takes up the drug which is quickly reduced to an unidentified polar product

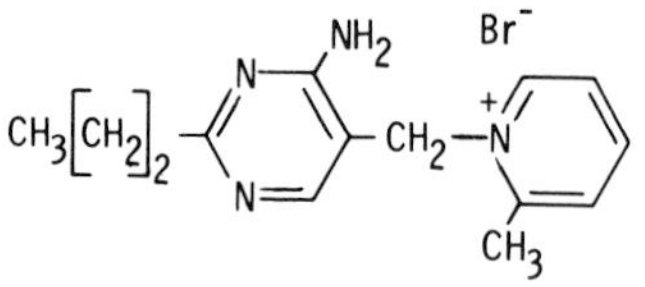

Amprolium

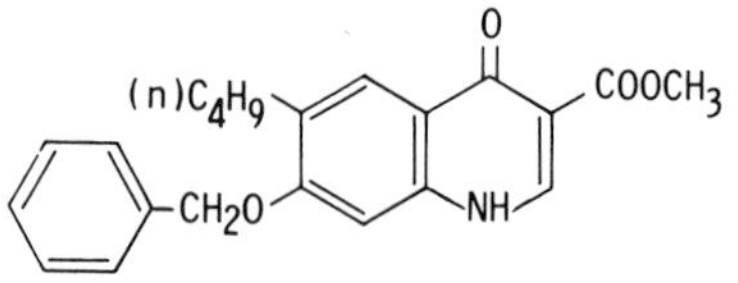

Methyl benzoquate

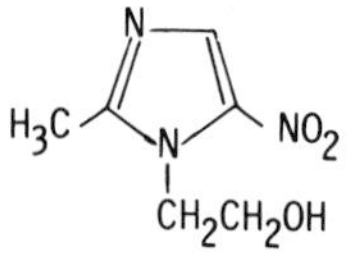

Metronidazole

Figure 6.10 Compounds used in the treatment of protozoal infections.

lacking the nitro group. The difficulties in defining the exact mode of action of this compound are similar to those experienced with the nitrofurans, as discussed above. Its activity is probably due to an unstable reduction product.

Chemotherapy of virus diseases

The success of drugs in the treatment of bacterial infections contrasts strongly with the meagre returns from the search for compounds active against virus infections. This is not surprising in view of the difference in the way these agents multiply in the body. Bacteria grow independently and have their own peculiar metabolic characteristics which provide points of selective attack. Virus infection and reproduction is a complex process which presents possibilities for interference at various stages from the initial binding of the infectious particle to the cell surface to the final liberation of newly synthesized virus. But since the process is essentially a subversion of normal cell metabolism the changes involved are subtle. Thus it is difficult to find compounds which will prevent virus production without damaging some vital cell mechanism.

Despite enormous efforts very few compounds are currently accepted as having a useful effect against diseases caused by viruses.

The antiviral agents 5-iododeoxyuridine and AraC (Fig. 4.20) have been discussed in Chapter 4. These cytotoxic agents are of considerable value in the treatment of herpes infections of the skin or eyes. More recently another nucleoside analogue, acyclovir (Fig. 6.11), has been developed. It seems to have little toxicity and shows considerable promise in the treatment of herpetic diseases. Amantadine (Fig. 6.11)

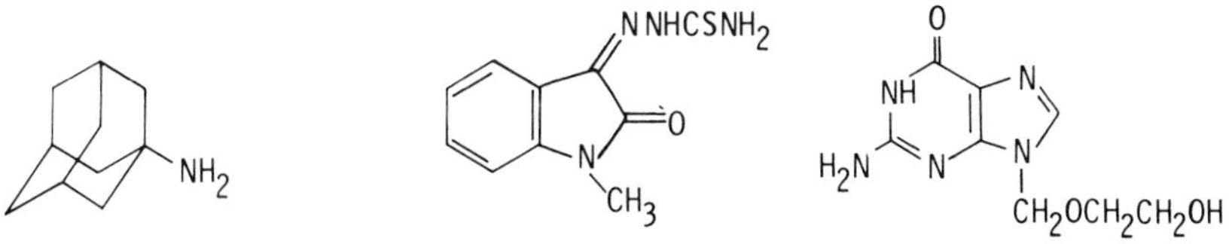

Figure 6.11 Compounds active against viruses.

has a specific prophylactic and curative effect against influenza A_2 infections in mice. In man it offers protection against influenza A_2 infection during the period of dosing, but curative action on the established disease is unproved. There is evidence that amantadine acts by preventing the penetration of the virus into the host cell; it may also inhibit the uncoating of the virus particle once it has entered the cell. Methisazone (Fig. 6.11) prevents the development of encephalitis in mice infected with various pox viruses. It was claimed to have prophylactic action in human smallpox, but since this disease has apparently been eliminated its use is irrelevant. Nevertheless its action is of interest. In Hela cells infected with vaccinia virus development is suppressed. The compound inhibits the synthesis of the protein required for encapsidation of the mature virus, the effect observed being a fragmentation of the mRNA produced late in virus development. There is no interference with the cell's normal protein synthesis.

Although the antiviral drugs now available are little used in clinical medicine, they serve to demonstrate that chemotherapy of virus infections is not, as some have thought, totally impracticable. Unfortunately they give few clues to ways of discovering new and more effective agents; this must still be regarded as a difficult and frustrating field of endeavour. Even where an active compound can be found, its action is likely to be restricted to a narrow class of viruses or even to a single strain. The main hope in the control of virus infections must rest with interferon. After 20 years of arduous research, sufficient supplies of human interferon should shortly become available to allow its potentialities to be tested widely. If its early promise is fulfilled, interferon will signal as great a victory in the therapy of virus diseases as the discovery of antibiotics achieved in the treatment of bacterial infections.

Further reading

Sulphonamides and dihydrofolate reductase inhibitors
G.H. HITCHINGS (1969), 'Chemotherapy and comparative biochemistry', in *Cancer Res.*, **29**, 1895.
M. FINLAND and E.H. KASS (eds) (1973), 'Trimethoprim-sulphamethoxazole' (Symposium), in *J. Infect. Dis.*, **128**, Supplement S425-S816.
S. ROLAND, R. FERONE, R.J. HARVEY, V.L. STYLES and R.W. MORRISON (1979), 'The characteristics and significance of sulphonamides as substrates for *Escherichia coli* dihydropteroate synthase', in *J. Biol. Chem.*, **254**, 10337.

Antimicrobial agents affecting terminal respiration
T.P. SINGER (1979), 'Mitochondrial electron-transport inhibitors', in *Methods Enzymol.*, **55**, 454.
E.C. SLATER (1973), 'The mechanism of action of the respiratory inhibitor antimycin', in *Biochim. Biophys. Acto.*, **301**, 129.
J.A. DOWNIE, F. GIBSON and G.B. COX (1979), 'Membrane adenosine triphosphatases of prokaryotic cells', in *Annu. Rev. Biochem.*, **48**, 103.
P.E. LINNETT and R.B. BEECHEY (1979), 'Inhibitors of the ATP synthetase system', in *Methods Enzymol.*, **55**, 472.

Compounds acting against mycobacteria
K. TAKAYAMA and L.A. DAVIDSON (1979), 'Antimycobacterial drugs that inhibit mycolic acid synthesis', in *Trends Biochem. Sci.*, **4**, 280.

Antifungal agents
M.R. SIEGEL and H.D. SISLER (eds) (1977), *Antifungal Compounds*, Vol. 1, Discovery, development and uses. Vol. 2, Interactions in biological and ecological systems (Marcel Dekker, 1977).
G.S. KOBAYASHI and G. MEDOFF (1977), 'Antifungal agents: recent developments', in *Annu. Rev. Microbiol.*, **31**, 291.
P.F. D'ARCY and E.M. SCOTT (1978), 'Antifungal agents' in *Drug Res.*, **22**, 93.

Antiprotozoal agents
W.E. GUTTERIDGE and G.H. COOMBS (1977), *Biochemistry of Parasitic Protozoa* (Macmillan, 1977).
H. VAN DEN BOSSCHE (1972), *Comparative Biochemistry of Parasites* (Academic Press, 1972).

Antiviral agents
D.L. SWALLOW (1978), 'Antiviral agents', in *Drug Res.*, **22**, 267.
C.E. HOFFMAN (1978), 'Antiviral agents', in *Annu. Rep. Med. Chem.*, **13**, 139.
R.J. WHITLEY and C.A. ALFORD (1978), 'Developmental aspects of selected antiviral chemotherapeutic agents', in *Annu. Rev. Microbiol.*, **32**, 285.

7 Penetrating the defences: how antimicrobial agents reach their targets

For a drug to inhibit the growth of a micro-organism it has to achieve an inhibitory concentration at its target site. The drug must first penetrate the various permeability barriers that separate the target site from the external environment. In the case of bacteria the differences in the properties of these permeability barriers among the various genera and species play an important role in determining the antibacterial spectrum of a drug. Target sites, e.g. ribosomes, DNA, enzymes etc., isolated from different groups of bacteria, are frequently found to be closely similar in sensitivity to an antibacterial agent and yet the intact cells have very different sensitivities. In many cases these variations in cellular sensitivities are due to differences in the composition of the bacterial cell envelopes which affect the ease of penetration of drugs to the target sites. The development of resistance to some antimicrobial agents depends upon a diminished permeability to the inhibitors. Sometimes the change in permeability is exquisitely selective, affecting only the movement of the inhibitor into the cell, and in other cases a generalized non-specific decrease in cellular permeability keeps the inhibitor out. The relationship of acquired drug-resistance to drug penetration is described in greater detail in Chapter 8.

Cellular permeability barriers to drug penetration

The cytoplasmic membrane

Common to all cellular micro-organisms is the permeability barrier provided by the cytoplasmic membrane. Its exact composition depends very much on the cell of origin but the most important feature is the lipid bilayer found in all cytoplasmic membranes. Drugs may cross this barrier either by passive diffusion or by facilitated diffusion involving a biological carrier system.

Passive diffusion

The rates of passive diffusion of uncharged organic molecules of molecular weight below 250 across lipid membranes correlate reasonably well with their lipid/water partition coefficients. That is, the more lipid-soluble a compound is, the more readily it enters and diffuses across the membrane. However, in a congeneric series of drugs, if the lipid solubility increases to a point where a drug is virtually insoluble in water, biological activity may decline sharply, presumably because the drug is reluctant to leave the lipid phase of the membrane for the watery environment of the cell interior. This phenomenon has been given mathematical expression in the 'Hansch equation' (so named after the scientist who formulated it):

$$\log (1/C) = -k(\log P)^2 + k'\log P + \rho\sigma + k''$$

where C is the molar concentration of the drug necessary to cause a standard biological response, in this case inhibition of cell growth and division, P is the partition coefficient, ρ and σ are physicochemical constants (Hammett constants) defining certain electronic features of the molecule and k, k' and k'' are empirically determined constants. The Hansch equation defines the parabolic relationship between the biological activity and the lipophilic character of a drug and in addition takes account of the electronic and structural features of the molecule. It indicates that in a chemically related series of biologically active drugs there is an optimal partition coefficient associated with maximum biological activity. It should be noted, however, that this relationship holds only for those agents which cross membranes by passive diffusion and it may be irrelevant when biologically facilitated transport of a drug is involved.

The Hansch equation has been applied to a wide range of sets of synthetic antibacterial compounds which penetrate the bacterial envelope by passive diffusion. The results show that compounds that are most active against Gram-negative bacteria are significantly less lipophilic than compounds highly active against Gram-positive organisms. The cytoplasmic membranes of the two classes of bacteria are sufficiently similar in total lipid content to make it unlikely that the differences in the partition coefficient of optimally active compounds could be explained by differences in the solvent properties of the cytoplasmic membranes. A more likely explanation is to be found in the different nature of the outer envelopes of Gram-negative and Gram-positive bacteria (Chapter 2). The greater lipid content of the Gram-negative outer envelope suggests that very lipophilic antibacterial agents would be retained in this fatty layer.

The abundant polysaccharide material that envelopes Gram-negative cells may also hinder the access of lipophilic drugs.

The rate of penetration across a lipid membrane by passive diffusion of water-soluble molecules of low lipid solubility is usually very slow. Small, i.e. molecular weight less than 100, un-ionized molecules move across as though the membrane were interspersed with water-filled channels or pores. These water-filled channels, which are presumed to exist in the cytoplasmic membrane, must be clearly distinguished from the larger well-defined hydrophilic pores in the outer membrane of Gram-negative bacteria (Chapter 2). While water-soluble antibiotics of molecular weight up to 600 or so pass through the pores of the outer membrane, their molecular size would preclude them from using the water-filled channels of the cytoplasmic membrane. Nevertheless, as we shall see, some large water-soluble antibiotics do enter bacterial cytoplasm with considerable facility.

Ionized water-soluble molecules of molecular weight greater than 100 are virtually unable to cross cytoplasmic membranes by passive diffusion. This is because ionized molecules in aqueous solution possess a strongly bound hydration shell, and only the very smallest ions can diffuse across membranes via the watery channels. The effect of ionization on the activity of an antibacterial agent is well illustrated by erythromycin. The pK_a of the basic group of this antibiotic is 8.8 and the concentration required for antibacterial activity decreases markedly as the pH of the bacterial medium is increased towards 8.8. Very likely only the un-ionized form of erythromycin penetrates into the bacteria and this represents an increasing proportion of the total erythromycin as the pK_a of the drug is approached.

Facilitated diffusion

A remarkable feature of cytoplasmic membranes is their ability to transfer certain physiologically important molecules across the membranes at rates very much higher than could occur by passive diffusion. This process, which is especially noticeable with water-soluble and ionized permeants, is known as facilitated transfer or facilitated diffusion. Characteristically, the rate of transfer of the permeant is proportional to its concentration over a limited range beyond which a limiting rate is approached. This is generally attributed to the involvement in the transfer process of carrier molecules specific for each permeant. Evidently the rate of transfer increases with increasing permeant concentration until all of the carrier sites are saturated. Facilitated diffusion, can therefore, usually be distinguished from passive diffusion, as in the latter process the transfer rate is proportional to the permeant concentration over a much wider range. Facilitated transfer by itself results in the equilibration of the permeant across the membrane. In some instances, however, when the transfer system is linked to an input of 'energy' the permeant may be transferred across the membrane against its concentration gradient. This phenomenon is known as 'active transport'. Facilitated transfer systems frequently show a high degree of specificity and only close structural analogues of the natural permeant compete effectively for the transport sites. From this we would expect facilitated transfer and active transport to be significant modes of penetration into micro-organisms only for those drugs whose chemical structures resemble natural cellular nutrients. This is generally borne out by experience, although there are a few examples (see below) of drugs not obviously resembling known nutrients that apparently gain access to their target sites by facilitated transfer mechanisms.

The outer layers of bacterial cells

Although the cytoplasmic membrane is a most important barrier against the penetration of many water-soluble antimicrobial chemicals, it is unlikely to provide the basis for the marked specificity of action of some antibiotics. Table 7.1 lists a number of agents that are active against both Gram-positive and Gram-negative bacteria and also several that are significantly active only against Gram-positive organisms. The poor activity of this second group of drugs against Gram-negative bacteria is almost certainly due to difficulty in

Table 7.1 Differential sensitivity and permeability to typical antibacterial drugs

Drugs active against Gram-positives and Gram-negatives	*Drugs less active against Gram-negatives because of permeability barriers*
Tetracyclines	Benzyl penicillin (penicillin G)
Streptomycin and aminoglycosides	Methicillin
Albomycin	Macrolides
Sulphonamides	Lincomycin
D-Cycloserine	Rifamycins
Chloramphenicol	Fusidic acid
Phosphomycin	Vancomycin
Puromycin	Bacitracin
Many synthetic antiseptics	Novobiocin
Nitrofurans	Actinomycin D
Ampicillin and carbenicillin	
Cephaloglycin	

penetrating the complex outer layers of Gram-negative cells.

The structures of the cell envelopes of the two main bacterial groups are described in Chapter 2. In Gram-negative bacteria the thin peptidoglycan layer is probably not a serious obstacle to the entry of compounds, but the outer membrane presents a formidable permeability barrier to many antibacterial agents. Because of their strongly polar, predominantly negatively charged nature, the teichoic acids of Gram-positive cells may influence the penetration of ionized molecules. The interaction of positively charged compounds, such as streptomycin, with teichoic acid generates a localized, high concentration of drug in the envelope which may enable the drug to challenge the permeability barrier of the cytoplasmic membrane more effectively. In contrast, the entry of anionic molecules may be retarded by teichoic acid, although the exquisite sensitivity of many Gram-positive bacteria to penicillins which are organic anions suggests that the repulsive effect of teichoic acid cannot be very significant.

The first indication that the layers lying outside the cell membrane influence drug penetration came from studies with Gram-negative cells having defective envelopes. L-Forms of *Proteus mirabilis* were found to be 100 to 1000 times more sensitive than intact cells to erythromycin and several other macrolides. There was a less striking increase in sensitivity to other common antibiotics including streptomycin, chloramphenicol and the tetracyclines. In L-forms the peptidoglycan envelope is also defective so that the relative contributions of the various outer layers of intact bacteria in hindering antibiotic penetration was uncertain. Many other studies since have clearly demonstrated the importance of the outer membrane as a major permeability barrier.

Treatment of Gram-negative bacteria with the chelating agent ethylenediaminetetra-acetic acid (EDTA) releases 30-50 per cent of the surface lipopolysaccharide, probably by sequestering the divalent cations, Ca^{2+} and Mg^{2+}, that appear to stabilize the outer envelope. Gram-negative cells treated in this way become much more sensitive to a number of agents, including lysozyme and those antibiotics listed in Table 7.1 to which intact Gram-negative cells are intrinsically resistant. An enhanced uptake of several antibiotics into EDTA-treated cells has been noted and since the cytoplasmic membrane and peptidoglycan are hardly affected by this treatment, changes in the outer membrane and a loss of the associated lipopolysaccharide are believed to be largely responsible for the increased permeability and antibiotic sensitivity.

Further evidence that the lipopolysaccharide of Gram-negative cells is a major determinant of sensitivity to many antibacterial agents emerged from studies of mutants with altered lipopoly-saccharides. Mutants of *Escherichia coli* that are 'supersensitive' to novobiocin, spiramycin and actinomycin D have lipopolysaccharide that lacks phosphate diester bridges in its backbone structure and is deficient in glucose, galactose and heptose. The remarkably specific nature of the effects is evident in that the supersensitive mutants are no more sensitive to benzyl penicillin than is the wild-type strain. Mutants of *Salmonella minnesota* that are more sensitive to erythromycin, actinomycin D and bacitracin are more resistant than the wild-type to tetracycline. The envelope lipopolysaccharide of these mutants is also deficient in sugar elements. Increased drug-resistance as well as increased sensitivity is also found among envelope mutants of Gram-negative bacteria. Unfortunately the changes in the composition of the lipopolysaccharides are not very illuminating. For example, the lipopolysaccharide of ampicillin-resistant mutants of *Salmonella typhimurium* lacks rhamnose, abequose and mannose, while that of ampicillin-resistant *E.coli* is depleted of rhamnose, galactose and glucose. At present, the significance of the loss of these sugar elements to the apparently decreased permeability of the bacterial envelopes to ampicillin is uncertain.

Pore structure of outer membrane of gram-negative bacteria

The outer membrane of Gram-negative bacteria does not have the capacity for the facilitated diffusion of essential nutrients. However, recent studies have revealed a remarkable feature of the outer membrane that permits the rapid transit of certain water-soluble molecules. The 'matrix' proteins, referred to in Chapter 2, are arranged to form pores across the lipid bilayer of the outer membrane which enable hydrophilic molecules, of molecular weight up to 600-700, to move easily across the membrane. In general the permeability afforded by the pores is non-specific. Certain water-soluble antibiotics normally move freely through these pores, and mutations which adversely affect the matrix proteins decrease bacterial sensitivity to drugs that use the pores, such as chloramphenicol and the β-lactam antibiotic cephaloridine. Lipid-soluble compounds cross the outer membrane by passive diffusion through the lipid bilayer. Specific receptors exist in the outer membrane for high-molecular-weight essential nutrients, such as vitamin B_{12} and the iron-transporting sideramines and enterochelins. These receptors permit the penetration of the outer membrane by specific high-molecular-weight nutrients, although the mechanism involved is unknown. The sideromycin antibiotics (Chapter 6), which closely resembles the sideramines, exploit the sideramine receptor in order to cross the outer membrane. A mutation affecting the sideramine receptor (*tonA*) markedly increases cellular resistance to the sideromycin, albomycin.

Changes in the lipid components of the Gram-negative outer layers have been described in the *envA* mutant of *E.coli* which shows increased sensitivity to actinomycin D. R-Factor mediated resistance to penicillins and chloramphenicol (see Chapter 8) is depressed by the *envA* mutation. There is an increase in cellular permeability to many drugs in cells with the *envA* mutation. The effect of the *envA* mutation on R-factor mediated resistance to penicillins and chloramphenicol may be due to the increased rate of penetration of these drugs resulting in the overloading of the enzymic mechanisms for their inactivation. Changes in the lipid include an increase in palmitic acid and a decrease in phosphatidyl glycerol and $C_{18:1}$ fatty acid content. At present, though, the functional significance of this information is unknown.

The barrier function of the Gram-negative outer envelope is a major determinant of the extraordinary resistance of *Pseudomonas aeruginosa* to antibacterial drugs. This potentially dangerous pathogen, which can cause life-threatening infections of wounds and burns, can be very difficult to eliminate with antibiotics. The outer envelope of *Ps. aeruginosa* is easily disrupted by treatment with EDTA and its antibiotic sensitivity is markedly increased, although this effect of EDTA is not clinically applicable.

Some examples of modes of penetration of antibacterial agents

Passive diffusion

Drugs that probably cross the cytoplasmic membrane by passive diffusion include: nalidixic and oxolinic acids, trimethoprim, the sulphonamides, the nitrofurans and chloramphenicol.

In the case of chloramphenicol, there is, as previously mentioned, some evidence that its movement across the outer membrane of Gram-negative bacteria may require a normally functioning pore complex despite the rather hydrophobic nature of the drug. Intracellular binding of chloramphenicol is partially dependent on a source of energy in the medium. While this could indicate the existence of an energy-linked facilitated diffusion mechanism in the cyto-plasmic membrane, it more likely reflects the energy dependence of the continued synthesis of chloramphenicol-binding sites within the cell.

A number of important antibiotics apparently cross the cytoplasmic membrane by passive diffusion despite their unfavourable physical characteristics. Included in this group are bulky molecules that are partially or very water-soluble, such as the macrolides, the rifamycins, lincomycin, clindamycin and fusidic acid. Although diffusion across the cytoplasmic membrane may be very slow, appreciable binding of these drugs to their intracellular targets promotes a net inward flux until the binding sites are saturated. Provided that the rate of occupation of the target sites is not substantially exceeded by the rate of synthesis of new sites, inhibition of cell growth and division rapidly develops.

Facilitated diffusion

D-cycloserine

This antibiotic is a structural analogue of D-alanine (Chapter 2), and it enters bacterial cells by the transport system in the cytoplasmic membrane for D-alanine. In *Streptococcus faecalis* D- and L-alanine use the same transport mechanism and D-cycloserine competitively inhibits the uptake of both isomers. In *E.coli*, however, there are separate systems for D- and L-alanine transport and D-cycloserine is a rather more effective inhibitor of D-alanine transport. Kinetic measurements reveal that there are high- and low- affinity transport systems for D-alanine and D-cycloserine in *E.coli* and, at the minimal concentration of D-cycloserine (4 μM) that inhibits the growth of *E.coli*, the drug utilized principally the high-affinity transport system which has a K_m of 42 μM for D-cycloserine. The facilitated transport system for D-alanine is energy-coupled and results in the intracellular accumulation of D-alanine and D-cycloserine against their concentration gradients. This is an important observation because the concentrations of D-cycloserine that produce significant inhibition of L-alanine racemase and D-alanyl-D-alanine synthetase in cell-free preparations are high compared with the minimal growth-inhibiting concentration.

Tetracyclines

The discovery that the tetracyclines are actively transported into bacterial cells but not into mammalian cells provided an explanation for the specificity of action and general lack of toxicity of these drugs (Chapter 5). The absence of any obvious structural similarity between the tetracyclines and known transportable cell nutrients has precluded a straightforward explanation of how the drugs are taken up by bacteria. In Gram-negative bacteria the water-soluble tetracyclines cross the outer membrane via the pores constructed from the matrix proteins. The lipophilic derivative minocycline, however, appears to diffuse through the lipid phase rather than through the pores. The events in the cytoplasmic membrane that effect the marked intracellular accumulation of the tetracyclines are more obscure. Accumulation is coupled to the energy metabolism of the cells and can result in an intracellular concentration of tetracycline 20-30 times that of the external medium. Before the onset of the energy-dependent uptake of tetracyclines, there is an energy-independent phase of binding to the cells, which, while not directly associated with the antibiotic action of the drugs, is probably an essential prelude to active accumulation. Although tetracyclines probably cross the cytoplasmic membrane with the aid of a protein carrier, direct evidence for this is lacking. The penetration of the lipophilic compound minocycline into the cytoplasm may be qualitatively different from that of the water-soluble tetracyclines. As we shall see in Chapter 8, inhibition of the active transport of tetracyclines underlies the commonest form of resistance to these antibiotics.

Sideromycins

These complex antibiotics subvert bacterial transport of the iron-sequestering sideramines at two sites. In Gram-negative bacteria, the sideromycins traverse the outer membrane following their interaction with the specific sideramine-receptor protein. Transport of the sider-amines across the cytoplasmic membrane involves facilitated diffusion coupled to energy metabolism. The sideromycin antibiotics also subvert this system to gain access to the cytoplasm. The maximum intracellular concentration of the sideromycin, A22765, is about one hundredfold greater than that in the medium. The antibiotic is, however, extensively bound to intracellular sites, i.e. the apparent concentration may not represent 'free' drug. We cannot say at present therefore whether the intracellular concentration of A22765 is entirely due to active transport. Mutant organisms defective in the cytoplasmic membrane transport of sideramines are resistant to sideromycin antibiotics, thus providing further evidence for the involvement of the sideramine-transport system in the accumulation of sideromycins.

Streptomycin

This water-soluble, ionized molecule presumably penetrates the outer membrane of Gram-negative bacteria via the pore system. Initial uptake into *E.coli* is characterized by a rapid electrostatic interaction between the positively charged guanidine groups of streptomycin and anionic residues located between the outer membrane and the cytoplasmic membrane. This is followed by a slow penetration of the antibiotic into the cytoplasm by an unknown mechanism. After 10 to 20 min a third phase of uptake begins which depends on a membrane-mediated, energy-linked process that results in intracellular accumulation of streptomycin. There is little doubt that the third phase of uptake depends on the synthesis of a permease induced by streptomycin itself. The initial binding of streptomycin to the ribosomes that occurs during the second phase of uptake initiates the synthesis of the permease. Mutants with ribosomes resistant to streptomycin fail to synthesize the permease. Gene activity is involved in permease induction as mutants with an impaired ability to express inducible operons have a greatly reduced permease response to streptomycin. As might be expected, the permease responsible for the third phase of streptomycin uptake is not concerned solely with antibiotic uptake but is in fact a physiological polyamine-transport system. Induction of this permease by streptomycin enhances cellular accumulation of spermidine and putrescine. There is competitive antagonism between polyamine and streptomycin uptake, indicating that these compounds share the same permease. Enhanced streptomycin uptake is induced by other aminoglycosides including kanamycin, gentamicin and neomycin, although not by spectinomycin. Although these findings were made with *E.coli*, it is likely that the mechanism of streptomycin uptake is widespread, at least in Gram-negative bacteria. Anaerobic bacteria probably owe their resistance to streptomycin and other aminoglycosides to an inability to accumulate these antibiotics.

Phosphomycin

This simple, phosphorus-containing antibiotic uses two different physiological transport systems to gain access to the bacterial cytoplasm. (i) The permease for α-glycerophosphate, which phosphomycin structually resembles. The ability of phosphomycin to use this permease is competitively antagonized by high concentrations of α-glycerophosphate. (ii) The permease for hexose 6-phosphates in certain enterobacteriacae and staphylococci can also be exploited by phosphomycin. Both these transport systems are induced by their physiological substrates, although not by phosphomycin. In an experimental infection with *E.coli* in mice, the therapeutic efficacy of phosphomycin is enhanced by pretreatment of the animals with glucose 6-phosphate. This effect can be attributed to the induction of the permease in the infecting cells permitting a higher intracellular concentration of phosphomycin.

The exploitation of transport systems in the design of new antimicrobial agents

The barrier function of the microbial cell provides both problems and opportunities for the designers of new drugs. In Gram-negative cells the outer membrane will be more easily breached by compounds that can utilize the pore system. Other specific nutrient receptors in the outer membrane may await discovery and eventual exploitation. A closer examination of the permeability characteristics of the outer envelope of *Ps.aeruginosa* might prove especially rewarding in the design of new agents to combat this troublesome pathogen.

The discovery of relatively non-specific permeases for small peptides in bacteria and other micro-organisms led to the demonstration that poorly permeating toxic amino acid analogues have enhanced antibacterial activity when attached to small peptides. The oligopeptide permease of *E.coli* recognizes and transports small peptides with up to 6 or 7 amino acids, although the molecular-sieving action of the outer membrane pores imposes a limit on the maximum molecular size of peptide that the intact organism can absorb. A free *N*-terminus is essential for peptide transport, but a variety of carboxyl-substituted peptides are accepted by the permease. Small toxic substituents at the *C*-terminus can therefore be 'smuggled' into the cell. An interesting example of a synthetic peptide analogue that exploits peptide permease is alaphosphin (Fig. 7.1). This compound, in which the carboxyl residue is replaced by a phosphonic acid group, is rapidly accumulated by *E.coli* to an intracellular concentration 100-1000 times that in the medium. The

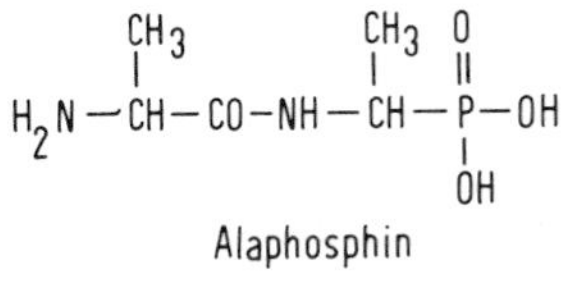

$$\underset{\text{H}_2\text{N}}{} -\text{CH}-\text{CO}-\text{NH}-\underset{\overset{\displaystyle \text{CH}_3}{|}}{\text{CH}}-\overset{\overset{\displaystyle \text{O}}{\|}}{\underset{\underset{\displaystyle \text{OH}}{|}}{\text{P}}}-\text{OH}$$

Alaphosphin

Figure 7.1 Alaphosphin or L-alanyl-L-1-amino-ethylphosphonic acid: a new antibacterial drug that exploits the peptide permease systems of bacterial cells to gain access to its intracellular target enzyme.

Table 7.2 Structural features in the bacterial cell envelope that influence the penetration of antibacterial agents

Structure	Effects on penetration
Polysaccharides of Gram-negative outer membrane	Retard or prevent penetration of many bulky, high-molecular-weight antibiotics, e.g. novobiocin, erythromycin
Lipid bilayer of Gram-negative outer membrane	Rate of penetration generally dependent on lipophilicity of solute, i.e. penetration of water-soluble drugs is severely hindered
Hydrophilic pores of Gram-negative outer membrane	Permit rapid penetration through outer membrane of water-soluble molecules up to 650 daltons in molecular size
Nutrient receptor proteins of Gram-negative outer membrane	Ensure penetration through outer membrane of higher-molecular-weight agents closely related to natural nutrients, e.g. sideromycins utilize sideramine receptor
Teichoic and teichuronic acids of Gram-positive bacteria	Strongly anionic character of these polymers may affect rate of penetration of ionized molecules
Lipid bilayer of cytoplasmic membrane	Rate of penetration generally dependent on lipophilicity of solute, i.e. penetration of water-soluble drugs is hindered
Nutrient transport proteins of cytoplasmic membrane	Facilitate rapid penetration of agents structurally related to natural nutrients, e.g. COOH-substituted peptides, D-cycloserine, phosphomycin. May also permit penetration of tetracyclines

energy-dependent accumulation requires L-L sterochemistry in the dipeptide. Inside the cell, alaphosphin is cleaved by aminopeptidase action to relase L-l-aminoethylphosphonic acid which inhibits alanine racemase and consequently the biosynthesis of the peptidoglycan of the bacterial wall (cf. D-cycloserine, Chapter 2). Alaphosphin shows activity against infections in man, although its place in medicine remains to be established.

Fungal infections are frequently refractory to conventional antibiotic therapy; in some instances this is due to the limited penetration of antibiotics into the cells. However, synergism has been observed between a number of antifungal agents and the polyene, amphotericin B. Presumably the polyene assists the penetration of impermeant inhibitors by disorganizing the cytoplasmic membrane. Since facilitated transport of peptides also occurs in fungi, it is possible that this could be exploited to introduce inhibitory molecules into fungal cells.

The influence of the major structures of bacterial cell envelopes on the penetration of antibacterial agents is summarized in Table 7.2

Further reading

General
W.D. STEIN (1967), *The movement of molecules across cell Membranes* (Academic Press, 1967).
W.N. KONINGS (1977), 'Active transport of solutes in bacterial membrane vesicles', in *Adv. Microb. Physiol.*, 15, 175.
M.S. TUTE (1971), 'Principles and practice of Hansch analysis: a guide to structure-activity correlation for the medicinal chemist', in *Adv. Drug Res.*, 6, 1.
T.J. FRANKLIN (1974), 'Factors affecting the penetration of antibiotics into bacteria', in *Ind. Asp. Biochem., Proc. 9th Meet. FEBS.*, 30, 549.
J.W. PAYNE (1977), 'Transport and hydrolysis of peptides by micro-organisms', in *Peptide Transport and Hydrolysis; Ciba Found. Symp.*, 50, 305.

The barrier function of the Gram-negative envelope
J.M. Di RIENZO, K. NAKAMURA and M. INOUYE (1978), 'The outer membrane proteins of Gram-negative bacteria: biosynthesis, assembly and functions', in *Annu. Rev. Biochem.*, 47, 481.
H. NIKAIDO and T. NAKAE (1979), 'The outer membrane of Gram-negative bacteria', in *Adv. Microb. Physiol.*, 20, 163.
M.R.W. BROWN (1975), 'The role of the cell envelope in resistance', p. 71, in *'Resistance of Pseudomonas aeruginosa'* ed. M.R.W. Brown, (John Wiley & Sons, 1975).
R.A. SCUDAMORE, T.J. BEVERIDGE and M. GOLDNER (1979), 'Outer-membrane penetration barriers as components of intrinsic resistance to Beta-lactam and other antibiotics in *Escherichia coli K12*', in *Antimicrob. Agents Chemother.*, 15, 182.

Antibiotic-transport mechanisms
I. CHOPRA and T.G.B. HOWE (1978), 'Bacterial resistance to the tetracyclines', in *Microbiol. Rev.*, 42, 707.
J.V. HÖLTJE (1978), 'Streptomycin uptake via an inducible polyamine system in *Escherichia coli*', in *Eur. J. Biochem.*, 86, 345.
F.M. KAHAN, J.S. KAHAN, P.J. CASSIDY AND H. KROPP (1974), 'The mechanism of action of fosfomycin (phosphonomycin), in *Ann. N.Y. Acad. Sci.*, 245, 364.
J.G. ALLEN, F.R. ATHERTON, M.J. HALL, C.H. HASSALL, S.W. HOLMES, R.W. LAMBERT, L.J. NISBET and P.S. RINGROSE (1978), 'Phosphonopeptides, a new class of synthetic antibacterial agents', in *Nature (London)*, 272, 56.

8 The problems of resistance to antimicrobial drugs

The development of safe, effective antimicrobial drugs has revolutionized medicine in the last forty years. Morbidity and mortality from microbial disease have been drastically reduced by modern chemotherapy. Unfortunately, micro-organisms are nothing if not versatile, and the brilliance of the chemotherapeutic achievement has been somewhat dimmed by the emergence of microbial strains presenting a formidable array of defences against growth-inhibiting drugs. This should not surprise us, of course, since the evolutionary history of living organisms is concerned with their adaptation to the environment. The eventual adaptation of micro-organisms to the toxic hazards of antimicrobial drugs is therefore probably inevitable.

The first detailed account of microbial drug-resistance was given by Paul Ehrlich in 1907 when he encountered this problem shortly after the development of arsenical chemotherapy against trypanosomiasis. Bacterial resistance appeared against the sulphonamides and against the antibiotics as these agents were brought into medical and veterinary practice. Microbial resistance to growth-inhibiting drugs is thus a widespread phenomenon and constitutes an ever-present threat to the successful treatment of infectious disease.

Our intention in this chapter is to give an outline of the genetic background to the problem of drug-resistance and then to describe the general types of biochemical mechanism that give rise to resistance. We shall draw upon a number of important examples of drug-resistance to illustrate these underlying biochemical mechanisms.

The genetics of drug-resistance

The tremendous advances made in the science of bacterial genetics over the past 35 years have found a most important practical application in furthering our understanding of the problem of drug-resistance. As a result we now have a farily complete picture of the genetic factors underlying the emergence of drug-resistant bacterial populations.

The early studies on the genetics of drug-resistance, however, were bedevilled by an exhausting controversy. On the one hand were those who believed that the development of a resistant cell population could be largely explained by phenotypic adaptation of the cells to an inhibitory compound without necessarily any significant modification in their genotype. The opposing faction took the view that any large population of cells which overall was sensitive to a drug was likely to contain small numbers of genotypically resistant cells. The continued presence of the drug resulted in the emergence of a new population of resistant cells by a process of selection.

Evidence gathered over the years strongly supports the second of these two theories. As we shall see, there are examples of phenotypic adaptation of bacterial cells to growth-inhibitory drugs; however, such cells are always genotypically different from the sensitive cells and generally do not constitute the majority of a wild-type population not previously exposed to the drug.

If the selective pressure applied by an antimicrobial drug is removed, a previously resistant microbial population often reverts eventually to the drug-sensitive phenotype. Sometimes the resistant cells are at a selective disadvantage to drug-sensitive cells in a drug-free environment and are therefore eventually outgrown by the sensitive cells. In other examples of reversion, the genetic material that confers drug-resistance is lost from the cells and the drug-resistant cells are progressively diluted out of the population.

The nature of genetic alterations that give rise to drug-resistant variants

Spontaneous mutations

Gene mutations are said to be spontaneous when they occur unprovoked by experimental mutagenic procedures. Spontaneous mutations occur with low frequency, i.e. one gene mutation per 10^5 to 10^7 cells per cell division. However, when the vast numbers of cells involved in bacterial populations are considered, the probability of a mutation arising in a gene causing a change from drug-sensitivity to drug-resistance is quite high. The simple and elegant technique of replica plating gives a convincing demonstration that spontaneous mutations to drug-resistance regularly occur in sensitive populations in the absence of the drug against which resistance develops (Fig. 8.1). Resistance is occasionally acquired by a cell in one large step, from sensitivity to high-level resistance, involving a mutation at a single locus. More frequently resistance results from a series of small, discrete steps involving successive mutations at multiple loci. In the second case highly resistant cells emerge only after prolonged or repeated exposure of the cell population to the drug.

Originally it was believed that the modifications of the genome by spontaneous mutation to drug-resistance, followed by the selection of resistant cells in the presence of drug, provided a satisfactory explanation for the emergence of drug-resistance populations. However, the discovery that bacterial cells can acquire additonal genetic material by the processes of transformation, transduction and conjugation led to the realization that spontaneous mutations may make only a minor contribution to the clinical problem of drug-resistance.

Spread of drug-resistance by the transfer of genetic information

Transformation

The discovery that DNA is the effective agent in the transforming principle from pneumococci was one of the most significant events in modern biology. Eventually it was found that the property of drug-resistance could be transferred *in vitro* to sensitive cells by treating them with DNA extracted from drug-resistant mutants. Since transformation of the morphological characteristics of pneumococcal colonies from smooth to rough forms can occur *in vivo* in infected animals, it is conceivable that transformation of sensitive cells to resistant could also occur *in vivo*. However, it should be remembered that transformation is a relatively inefficient way of spreading genetic information, since for each resistance marker acquired by a sensitive cell, a resistant cell must lyse in order to release its DNA. A somewhat more favourable situation may be envisaged where resistance is determined by multiple genetic loci. Then resistance is transformed into sensitive cells by unit steps each conferring partial resistance. Thus, a number of recipient cells might acquire bits of DNA derived from a single cell, each conferring partial drug-resistance. Despite this consideration, however, genetic transformation probably does not contribute substantially to the clinical problem of drug-resistance.

Transduction

During the process of phage transduction, which occurs in both

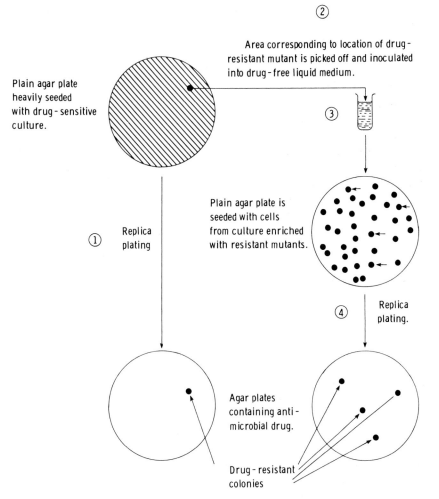

Figure 8.1 The technique of replica plating reveals the existence of drug-resistant cells in a population that is overall drug-sensitive. A plain agar plate is heavily seeded with cells from the drug-sensitive culture, and is incubated until growth occurs. Cells are transferred by a velvet pad to a plate containing the antibacterial drug; this plate is then incubated and the position of any colonies is noted. The area on the drug-free plate corresponding to the location of the resistant colony on the drug plate is picked off and cultured in drug-free medium. Although still contaminated with sensitive cells, this culture will contain many more resistant cells that the original culture. Plating out of the 'enriched' culture on a plain plate followed by replication to a drug plate therefore reveals a higher incidence of drug-resistant colonies. The experiment indicates that drug-resistant mutants occur in a bacterial population not previously exposed to the drug.

Gram-positive and Gram-negative bacteria, genetic information is transferred by phage particles from one bacterial cell to a related, phage-susceptible cell. In lysogeny the DNA of the infecting temperate phage is inserted into the bacterial genome where it replicates synchronously with the bacterial DNA until the integrated temperate phage reproduces itself virulently either spontaneously or as a result of treatment with ultraviolet light or certain chemicals. Complete phage particles are produced and the bacterial cell is lysed. Before unrestricted replication of the phage DNA occurs it is first released from the bacterial chromosome. During this phase short stretches of the bacterial chromosome that were contiguous with the phage DNA in the integrated state may be carried with the phage DNA and subsequently replicated as part of the phage genome. A similar process can result in the acquisition by the phage of genetic material from bacterial plasmids, which are genetic elements capable of independent existence in bacterial cells separate from the chromosome. The reader is referred to a suitable text on bacterial genetics for a fuller discussion of the complexities of phage trans-duction. Nevertheless, it can be seen that a transducing phage might pick up a stretch of DNA containing a drug-resistance determinant from a resistant bacterium during the process of induction. Lysis of the cell releases multiple copies of the phage each carrying a copy of the drug-resistance marker. Subsequent infection of phage-susceptible, drug-sensitive cells under conditions favouring lysogeny results in the newly infected cells becoming drug-resistant. In some cases a drug-resistance determinant from the original host is incorporated into the phage particle only at the expense of part of the phage genome. The resulting defective phage, while conferring the property of drug-resistance on infected recipient cells, cannot enter the lysogenic state, i.e. it cannot be subsequently induced to lyse the cells. How-ever, provided that the phage DNA, together with the acquired resistance marker, replicates normally in the recipient cells, a clone of drug-resistant cells arises from each parent infected with a trans-ducing phage. The transduction of plasmid determinants of drug-resistance usually occurs with much greater facility than that of chromosomal determinants. Possibly this reflects the ability of plasmids to replicate in a variety of environments, whereas the replication of chromosomal DNA is closely adapted to a specific organism.

The spread of drug-resistance markers by transduction is of considerable significance in *Staphylococcus aureus*. This organism harbours plasmids which confer resistance to a number of important antibiotics including penicillin, chloramphenicol, tetracycline and erythromycin as well as resistance to certain toxic metals. If a trans-ducing phage is introduced into *S. aureus* containing plasmids that confer drug-resistance, the property of drug-resistance can then be transferred by a lysate of the cells to drug-sensitive *S. aureus*. There is some evidence that the transduction of drug-resistance plasmids occurs spontaneously during staphylococcal infections in animals. Moreover, the widespread occurrence of these plasmids in staphylo-cocci isolated from hospital sources strongly suggests that transduction is an important factor in the emergence of drug-resistant strains of staphylococci. Phage transduction may also be significant to the spread of drug-resistance among the streptococci.

Conjugation and R-factors

The spread of drug-resistance by cellular conjugation in Gram-negative bacteria harboured by animals and man is recognized as an important clinical threat to the treatment of diseases caused by Gram-negative organisms. The phenomenon of cell conjugation in Gram-negative bacteria was discovered some years before its importance in drug-resistance was appreciated.

The realization that drug-resistance could be transferred during cell conjugation came from combined epidemiological and bacterial genetic studies in Japan. The first clue was provided by the isolation, from patients suffering from dysentery, of strains of *Shigella* that were resistant to a number of drugs, including sulphonamides, streptomycin, chloramphenicol and tetracycline. Even more striking was the discovery that both sensitive and multi-resistant strains of *Shigella* could occasionally be isolated from the same patient in the same epidemic. Most patients harbouring multi-resistant *Shigella* also had multi-resistant *Escherichia coli* in the intestinal tract. This suggested that the drug-resistance markers might be transferred from *E. coli* to *Shigella* and vice versa. Subsequently it was found that Gram-negative bacteria can indeed transfer drug-resistance not only to cells of the same species but also to bacteria of different species or even different genera.

The bacterial plasmids that are associated with the transference of drug-resistance markers by cellular conjugation are called R-factors. Under most conditions they are quite separate from the bacterial chromosome. They consist of two distinct but frequently linked entities (Fig. 8.2): (a) the resistance transfer factor ('RTF'), some-times called the Δ factor, which initiates and controls the conjugation process; (b) a series of one or more linked genes that confer resistance to specific antibacterial agents. The RTF is

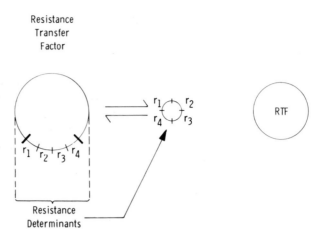

Resistance
Transfer
Factor

r_1 r_2
r_4 r_3

RTF

r_1 r_2 r_3 r_4

Resistance
Determinants

Figure 8.2 Diagrammatic representation of an R-factor and its reversible dissociation into two components. Although not shown in the diagram, if the R-factor carries a determinant for tetracycline-resistance this determinant almost certainly remains linked to the RTF after dissociation whereas the other resistance determinants r_1 r_2 r_3 r_4 ... r_n form a separate replicon.

analogous to the sex or F-factor which also confers on Gram-negative bacteria the ability to conjugate with cells lacking an F-factor. The complete R-factor resembles the F-prime factor (F′) in carrying genetic material additional to that which controls conjugation.

A bewildering variety of R-factors has been described carrying various combinations of drug-resistance determinants. Apart from the obvious property of drug-resistance, other phenotypic characteristics are conferred on the cells by different R-factors and these have prompted attempts to classify R-factors. The characteristics include: (i) The ability (fi^+) or inability (fi^-) to repress the fertility properties of an F-factor present in the same cell. (ii) The type of sex pilus (see below) that the R-factor determines. (iii) The inability of an R-factor to co-exist in a bacterium with certain other plasmids; this leads to the classification of R-factors into incompatibility groups. (iv) The presence of genes in the R-factor that specify DNA restriction and modification enzymes. An R-factor cannot be defined on the basis of a single characteristic, and a combination of properties must be used to classify it.

Transposons

Recent discoveries in molecular genetics provide a possible explanation for the very wide distribution of drug-resistance determinants among the plasmids and chromosomes of many bacterial species. For many years the transference of genes among plasmids and chromosomes was believed to occur as a result of a classical recombination mechanism dependent on the product of the bacterial *recA* gene and the reciprocal exchange of DNA in regions of considerable genetic homology. This permits the exchange of genetic information only between closely related genomes. Such a restricted phenomenon seemed unlikely to explain the widespread distribution of specific resistance determinants. It is now clear that the acquisition of genetic material by plasmids and chromosomes in bacteria is not limited by the classical *recA*-dependent recombination. Certain replicons, known as transposons, are able to insert themselves into a variety of genomic sites that have no common ancestry, i.e. homology, with the inserting sequence. In the simplest transposons the whole of the genetic information is concerned with the insertion function. More complex transposons contain additional genes that determine a variety of functions including resistance to antibiotics. Transposons have been found with resistance determinants for ampicillin, tetracycline, kanamycin, streptomycin, sulphonamides, chloramphenicol and trimethoprim. The biological significance of these complex transposons is that they facilitate the movement of resistance determinants between chromosomes, R-factors and phages. The widespread use of antibacterial drugs in medical and veterinary practice and in animal husbandry has encouraged the selection of bacterial plasmids with transposons. Almost certainly it is the traffic of transposons independent of *recA* that produces the accumulation of replicons with assemblies of genes conferring resistance to numerous antibiotics. The reader can explore the detailed complexities of transposons in a recent review referred to at the end of this chapter.

Molecular properties of R-factors

R-factors can be isolated from host bacteria as circular DNA (Fig. 8.3) in both closed and 'nicked' forms. There has been some debate as to the proportions of closed and nicked circles that arise during the isolation procedures. Nevertheless there is little doubt that both forms exist in the cell; the closed circular structure is probably adopted by R-factors when not engaged in replication. The contour lengths and thus molecular weights of isolated R-factors depend very much on the host bacterium and upon the culture conditions prevailing immediately before the isolation procedure. The R-factor may sometimes dissociate into two distinct components, the RTF and the resistance (r) determinant. This is more likely to occur in some host species, e.g. *Proteus mirabilis* and *Salmonella typhimurium*, than

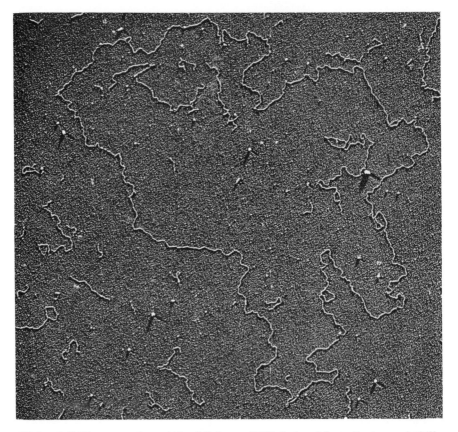

Figure 8.3 Electron micrograph of R-factor DNA isolated from *Proteus mirabilis* harbouring an R-factor with resistance markers to streptomycin, sulphonamides and chloramphenicol. The circular DNA molecule has a total length of 28.5 μm. This photograph is reproduced by kind permission of Dr Royston Clowes and the American Society for Microbioloty [*J. Bacteriol.*, 97 (1969) 383].

others, e.g. *E.coli*, where dissociation hardly ever occurs. The dissociation event seems to depend on the activity of a simple transposon that may be inserted at the junction of the RTF and the resistance determinant. Estimates of the molecular weights of RTFs from different R-factors lie between 50×10^6 and 60×10^6, with a buoyant density of 1.709. The molecular weight of the r-determinant depends on the number of drug-resistance genes carried, but typically it is much lower than that of the RTF. Thus an r-determinant carrying markers for resistance to chloramphenicol, streptomycin, spectinomycin and sulphonamide has a molecular weight of 12×10^6 with a buoyant density of 1.717.

The numbers of R-factors harboured by individual bacteria is influenced both by the properties of the plasmid and of its host as well as by the culture conditions. As a general rule (to which there are exceptions), the larger R-factors are present only in a limited number of copies (one to four) per chromosome in *E.coli*, whereas in *P. mirabilis* the number is much more variable and varies during the growth cycle. In stationary phase, replication of the R-factor continues for some time after chromosomal replication has ceased. Conditions that give rise to an increased number of R-factor copies are sometimes associated with enhanced resistance. However, the level of resistance does not always reflect the number of resistance gene copies. For example, although the number of R-factor copies is frequently greater in *P. mirabilis* than in *E.coli* the level of drug-resistance expressed in the former organism is usually lower than in *E.coli*. This is the case for resistance to several different antibiotics, and factors other than the number of gene copies may be more important in determining drug-resistance. Resistance-gene-dosage effects are not known to be significant in the treatment of bacterial infections.

The conjugation process

Cells bearing an R-factor (R^+) are characterized by the ability to produce surface appendages known as sex pili. The sex pili of R^+ bacteria closely resemble those produced by F^+ organisms. When 'male' R^+ cells are mixed with sensitive R^- 'female', mating pairs are immediately formed by some sort of surface interaction (Fig. 8.4) possibly involving the sex pili. The transfer of a copy of the R-factor from the R^+ to the R^- cell begins immediately and the acquisition of the R-factor by the 'female' cell converts it to a fertile, drug-resistant cell that can in turn conjugate with other R^- cells. In this way drug-resistance spreads rapidly through the bacterial population. Many of the fine details of the conjugation processes are still lacking, for example the role of the pilus in the transfer of plasmids is uncertain. Despite the attraction of the idea that the plasmid passes through the bore of the pilus, it is very difficult to prove directly. The significance of the replication of the R-factor DNA to the transfer process is also not clear. The R-factor copy is very likely transferred as a linear single-stranded molecule which is converted to a duplex immediately it gains access to a replication site in the recipient cell. Fortunatley perhaps, the frequency of R-factor transfer is much lower than that of F transfer. After infection of an R^- cell with an R-factor a repressor substance is thought to accumulate which eventually inhibits sex

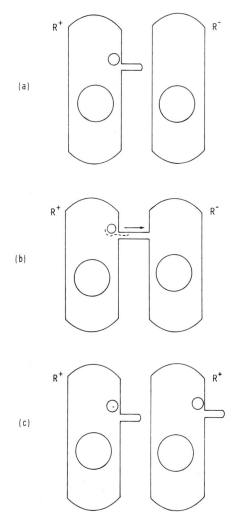

Figure 8.4 Diagrammatic representation of conjugation and transference of an R-factor in Gram-negative bacteria. a The chromosomes and R-factor are represented by large and small circles respectively, the solid lines indicating double-stranded DNA. b The mating pair is formed and a linear, single-stranded copy of the R-factor (broken line) may enter the pilus, which has formed a bridge between the partners, to gain entry to the R⁻ cell. c R-factor transfer is complete, the transferred single-stranded R-factor has converted to a duplex, circularized molecule and the bacterial partners separate. It should be noted that the role of the sex pilus in R-factor transfer as depicted in this diagram is still hypothetical.

pilus formation. The ability to conjugate is therefore restricted to a short period immediately after acquisition of the R-factor. Sex pilus production in F^+ cells, by contrast, is not under repressor control and conjugatory activity is therefore completely unrestricted. Mutant R-factors exist which have lost the ability to restrict sex pilus formation and the frequency of R-factor transfer among bacteria bearing this type of plasmid is much higher.

Clinical importance of R-factors

It is generally agreed that R-factors existed before the development of modern antibacterial drugs. Clearly though, the widespread use and abuse of these drugs have led to a vast increase in the incidence of drug-resistance caused by R-factors. This has been especially noticeable in farm animals such as chickens and pigs which in many countries until recently received clinically valuable antibacterial drugs in their foodstuffs as growth promoters. These animals acted as a reservoir for Gram-negative bacteria, such as *E.coli* and *Salmonella typhimurium*, harbouring R-factors potentially transferable to man. Fortunately, in some countries, strict controls have been imposed on the use as growth promoters of drugs valuable in human clinical medicine, resulting in a significant decline in the incidence in farm animals of R-factors mediating resistance to clinically important drugs.

The contribution of R-factor-bearing Gram-negative organisms to human morbidity and mortality is still uncertain. In human disease, however, an important example of the role of organisms bearing R-factor is the neonatal diarrhoea caused by certain pathogenic strains of *E.coli*. While the major requirement in the treatment of this distressing disease is the prevention of fatal dehydration, elimination of the pathogenic organisms may also be most important and this is often difficult in the event of multiple resistance to the commonly used antibacterial agents. In one notorious outbreak of this disease the children were infected with a pathogenic strain of *E.coli* resistant to penicillin, streptomycin, chloramphenicol, tetracycline, erythromycin, neomycin, novobiocin, cloxacillin and ampicillin. The infection eventually responded to gentamicin which was the only drug of those tested to which the pathogenic bacteria were sensitive. Another potentially alarming development has been the occasional appearance of *Salmonella typhi*, the causative organism of typhoid, with an R-factor-conferring resistance to chloramphenicol and cotrimoxazole, the drugs most commonly used to treat this disease.

Ecological features fortunately tend to limit the clinical threat posed by R-factors. Firstly the environment of the gastro-intestinal tract almost certainly depresses the conjugal activity of R^+ bacteria below that observed under ideal culture conditions in the laboratory. The emergence of an R^+ population of bacteria during antibiotic therapy is more likely to result from selection of resistant cells than from extensive conjugal transfer of resistance. After cessation of antibiotic treatment, the number of R^+ bacteria in the faeces declines; it seems that in the absence of drugs the colonizing ability of R^+ *E.coli* in the gut is lower than that of the normal R^- residents. R-factors do not themselves impair the colonizing ability of bacteria, but the organisms that preferentially harbour them tend to be poor colonizers.

Biochemical mechanisms of drug-resistance

Some years ago the American microbiologist Bernard Davis listed a number of possible mechanisms by which cells might resist the toxic effects of a growth-inhibiting drug. While this list continues to be useful, experience has shown that certain mechanisms of resistance are much more frequently encountered than others, at least in bacteria.

Summary of possible mechanisms

(1) Conversion of an active drug to an inactive derivative by enzyme(s) produced by the resistant cells.
(2) Modification of the drug-sensitive site.
(3) Loss of cell permeability to a drug.
(4) Provision of an alternative enzyme or pathway that bypasses the inhibited reaction.
(5) Increased levels of the enzyme inhibited by the drug.
(6) Increased concentration of a metabolite that antagonizes the inhibitor.
(7) Decreased requirement for a product of the inhibited metabolic system.

We shall illustrate these various mechanisms with appropriate examples and indicate their relative importance to the general problem of microbial resistance. However, it should be realized that the resistance of bacterial cells to an antibiotic may not depend on just one of these mechanisms. Especially in Gram-negative bacteria, resistance results both from the natural permeability barrier of the outer envelope that slows drug access and from more specific mechanisms of resistance that may inactivate a drug, prevents its transport across the cytoplasmic membrane or its binding to intracellular sites.

(1) Conversion of an active drug to an inactive derivative

Inactivation of β-lactam antibiotics

An important example of this type of resistance is the destruction of penicillin by bacteria that produce penicillinase (β-lactamase). The reaction (Fig. 8.5) involves the opening of the β-lactam bond of penicillin to give the inactive penicilloic acid. As we shall see later, the nature of the side chain, R, can be of critical importance in determining the susceptibility of the β-lactam bond to penicillinase. The related antibiotics, the cephalosporins, are also degraded by β-lactamase (Fig. 8.5). The immediate end product of cephalosporin degradation is cephalosporanoic acid, although this compound is so unstable that it spontaneously undergoes a complex series of degradative reactions. Penicillin and cephalosporin β-lactamases are

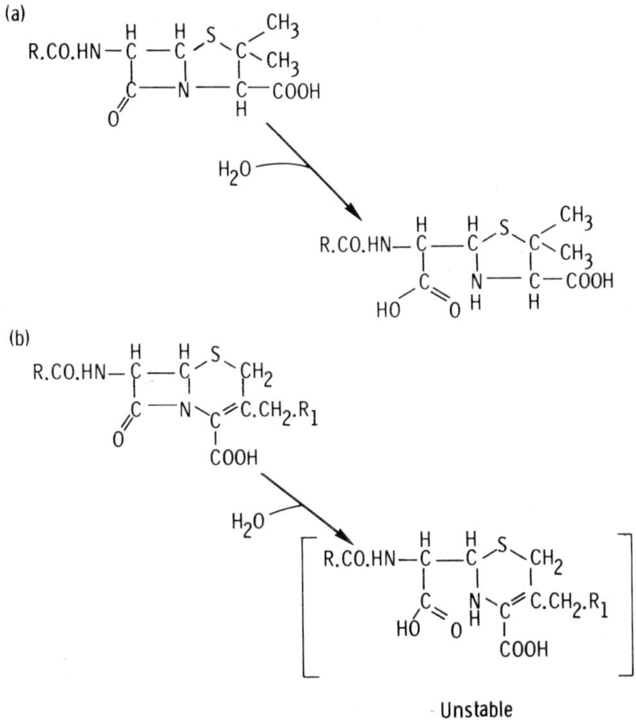

Figure 8.5 Inactivation of a penicillins and b cephalosporins by β-lactamase. In both cases the β-lactam bond is broken by a hydrolytic mechanism, but, whereas penicilloic acid is relatively stable, the corresponding cephalosporin product is highly unstable and decomposes spontaneously to a complex mixture. R and R_1 indicate variable side chains.

produced by many Gram-positive and Gram-negative bacteria. These enzymes are largely responsible for the high level of penicillin- and cephalosporin-resistance seen in Gram-positive bacteria that produce them. Particular enzymes often exhibit preferences for either penicillins or cephalosporins as substrates, so that cross-resistance between the two classes of β-lactam antibiotics is frequently incomplete.

The most important β-lactamase in Gram-positive bacteria is that produced by *S. aureus* which was responsible for the alarming rise in the resistance of this pathogen to penicillin that occurred in the late 1940s. and the 1950s. The β-lactamase of *S. aureus* is an inducible enzyme. The production of the enzyme is very low in the absence of penicillin or cephalosporin. When the β-lactamase gene is depressed by the addition of minute quantities of antibiotic (as little as $0.0024/\mu g/ml$ of medium) enzyme production is so greatly increased that it may account for more than 3 per cent of the total protein being synthesized by the bacterium. The enzyme is released from the bacterial cell and inactivates the antibiotic in the surrounding medium. Considerable dilution of β-lactamase occurs and this is the source of the observed 'inoculum effect'. In a small inoculum the few cells have no chance of destroying all of the surrounding antibiotic, but in an inoculum containing many cells, the concerted production and release of β-lactamase can contain the challenge. Staphylococcal resistance to penicillin is therefore very dependent upon inoculum size.

The β-lactamase of *S. aureus*, which has a molecular weight of approximately 29 000, is related in its amino acid sequence to the inducible β-lactamases of *Bacillus licheniformis* and *Bacillus cereus*. In *S. aureus* the gene for β-lactamase usually occurs on a plasmid which may also carry markers for resistance to other antibiotics. The clinical problem posed by staphylococcal resistance due to β-lactamase has been largely overcome by the development of novel semi-synthetic penicillins and cephalosporins that are poor substrates for β-lactamase and yet retain excellent antibiotic activity (see below).

Gram-negative β-lactamases

The nature of Gram-negative resistance to β-lactam antibiotics differs considerably from that of Gram-positive bacteria. The complex outer envelope of Gram-negative cells makes them intrinsically less sensitive to the original β-lactam antibiotics. However, soon after the appearance of semi-synthetic broad-spectrum compounds, such as ampicillin, resistance in Gram-negative pathogens that was evidently due to β-lactamase activity began to emerge. Since those early days an extraordinary number of β-lactamases has been discovered in Gram-negative bacteria. So many in fact that it has proved difficult to devise ways of classifying them. The Gram-negative β-lactamases fall broadly into two groups: (1) Enzymes determined by chromosomal genes. In many genera these enzymes are inducible by β-lactams. (2) Enzymes determined by plasmid genes on R-factors. Plasmid-mediated β-lactamases are produced constitutively in small amounts and remain bound to the cells. They therefore hinder the access of intact β-lactams to the membrane-associated target sites by destroying the antibiotics within the cell envelope, perhaps largely in the periplasmic space.

The Gram-negative β-lactamases can be further subdivided on the basis of their activities against penicillins, cephalosporins and the many semi-synthetic variants of these molecules. Most chromosomally-mediated β-lactamases inactivate both cephalosporins and penicillins, being considerably more active against the former group. Chromosomal enzymes specific for penicillins are exceedingly rare. By far the most important R-factor-mediated β-lactamase is the TEM-1 enzyme which has a broad activity range against penicillins and cephalosporins. The wide distribution of TEM-1 almost certainly results from the gene for this enzyme being carried on a transposon (Tn4). The closely related enzyme, TEM-2, is less widely distributed than TEM-1.

Chemical approaches to the β-lactamase problem

The advent of the semi-synthetic β-lactams during the 1950s offered an escape from the problem of bacterial resistance caused by β-lactamase. Compounds such as methicillin and cloxacillin (Chapter 2) that have bulky substituents in the penicillin side chain were found to be poor substrates for β-lactamase. The affinity of methicillin for staphylococcal β-lactamase is much lower than that of benzyl penicillin, and the maximum rate of hydrolysis of methicillin by this enzyme is only one-thirtieth of that of benzyl penicillin. Methicillin is an effective drug against infections caused by β-lactamase-producing staphylococci, even though its intrinsic anti-bacterial activity is substantially lower than that of benzyl penicillin. Although methicillin is only slowly degraded by Gram-negative β-lactamases, the drug is not effective against Gram-negative infections, as it fails to penetrate the outer envelope of these organisms. To combat the menace of Gram-negative β-lactamases, therefore, compounds were needed that both resisted β-lactamase attack and penetrated to the target sites in the cytoplasmic membrane. The substituted cephalosporins undoubtedly go a long way towards satisfying these requirements. Compounds such as cefuroxime, cefoxitin and HR756 (Chapter 2) combine good intrinsic activity against Gram-negative pathogens and considerable stability to the major β-lactamases.

The use of inhibitors of β-lactamases is an alternative approach to the control of resistant organisms that has received considerable attention in recent years with the discovery of several powerful, inhibitors. Methicillin, for example, is a fairly effective inhibitor of certain β-lactamases, and by protecting lactamase-susceptible compounds from inactivation methicillin can give a synergistic inhibitory effect when used in combination with other β-lactams. Unfortunately, this effect is of little clinical use. The discovery of the naturally occurring inhibitor, clavulanic acid (Fig 2.14), has dramatically opened the way for clinically valuable synergism with β-lactamase-susceptible agents such as ampicillin. Clavulanic acid, unlike methicillin, has little antibiotic activity of its own but it is a remarkably effective inhibitor of the β-lactamases of Gram-positive and Gram-negative bacteria. Since clavulanic acid contains a β-lactam ring, the compound most probably attacks β-lactamase at or near its active centre to produce a covalently bonded complex that is only slowly cleaved to release active enzyme. Clavulanic acid, therefore, behaves rather like a substrate with a low Michaelis constant but also with a very low V_{max}. This discovery has prompted a wide search for other inhibitors of β-lactamases, and it is likely that such compounds will enter medical practice to extend the usefulness of highly active β-lactamase-susceptible drugs.

Origin of β-lactamases

There is ample evidence that pencillin- and cephalosporin-destroying enzymes existed in bacteria long before the development of these antibiotics by medical science. The widespread and often indiscriminate use of the penicillins has certainly encouraged an alarming rate of spread of resistant bacteria but at least clinical usage cannot be held responsible for the existence of the β-lactamases. If antibiotics, such as penicillin and cephalosporins, are released under natural conditions from the micro-organisms that produce them, the synthesis of β-lactamases by other organisms sharing the same micro-environment might be regarded as the result of a long evolutionary process directed by the selected pressure of the antibiotics. However, difficulty in demonstrating the actual secretion of antibiotics under natural conditions casts some doubt on the survival value of antibiotics to micro-organisms and therefore on the selective advantage of enzymes such as the β-lactamases. It has been suggested that β-lactamase may have a physiological role apart from that of the inactivation of the β-lactam antibiotics; there may be a natural, physiological substrate other than these antibiotics, although the existence of this substrate has yet to be convincingly demonstrated.

An alternative suggestion is that β-lactamases may be the product of a mutant form of one of the genes coding for the penicillin/cephalosporin target enzymes, i.e. the transpeptidases involved in the final cross-linking stage of peptidoglycan biosynthesis and D-alanine carboxypeptidase (Chapter 2). β-Lactams form covalent complexes with these enzymes, but, although the complexes are usually sufficiently stable to ensure inhibition of peptidase function, there is evidence that in some cases the enzymes act as inefficient β-lactamases. True β-lactamases might have resulted from an evolutionary process that markedly enhanced the β-lactamase function at the expense of the original transpeptidase activity. At some early stage there must have been duplication of a transpeptidase gene in order that the organism should retain the capacity for normal cell wall synthesis while evolving β-lactamase activity from mutations in the other gene copy.

Inactivation of chloramphenicol by acetylation

Another important example of bacterial drug-resistance due to inactivation of the antibiotic is the enzymic acetylation of chloramphenicol by resistant strains of both Gram-positive and Gram-negative bacteria. Chloramphenicol-resistant strains of *S. aureus,* carrying the resistance marker on an extrachromosomal plasmid, and also *E.coli*, carrying the chloramphenicol-resistance determinant on an R-factor, both destroy the antibiotic properties of the drug. Possibly the widespread occurrence of this type of resistance to chloramphenicol is due to the occurrence of a gene for chloramphenicol-resistance on a transposon (Tn9). It depends whether this transposon proves to be common among plasmids or whether it is peculiar to those transducing phages on which it is found. Cell-free extracts of resistant strains convert chloramphenicol to the 3-acetoxy and 1, 3-diacetoxy derivatives provided that adequate amounts of acetyl-coenzyme A (acetyl-CoA) are present (Fig. 8.6). Corresponding extracts from chloramphenicol-sensitive bacteria cause no significant acetylation. Very recently, several new derivatives of chloramphenicol have been described which are not subject to acetylation and yet retain antibacterial activity. The

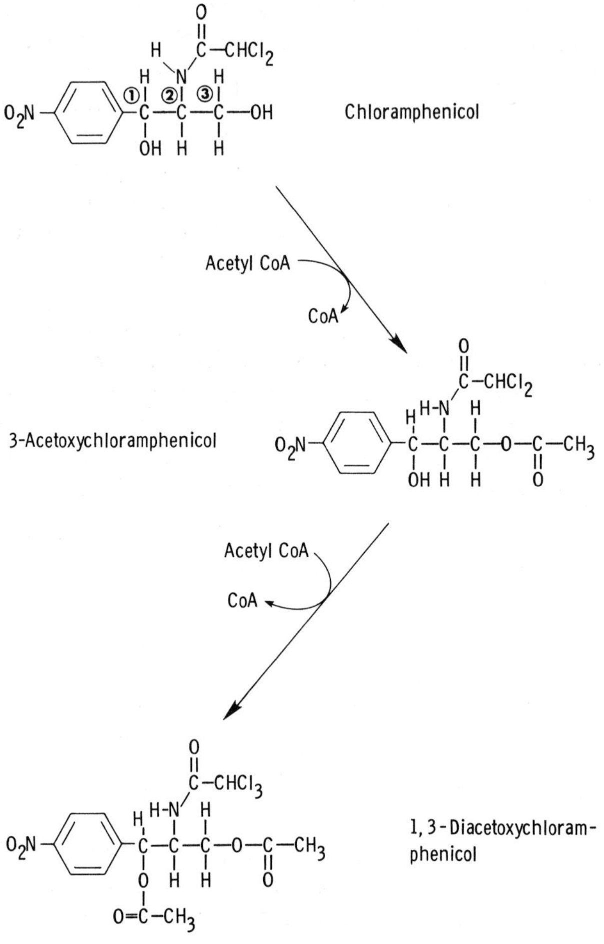

Figure 8.6 Inactivation of chloramphenicol by chloramphenicol acetyl transferase; 3-acetoxychloramphenicol is formed first and 1,3-diacetoxychloramphenicol probably forms by a non-enzymic shift of the acetyl group to the 1-position followed by acetylation of the free 3-OH group.

key substitution appears to be the replacement of the *terminal* OH group of the side chain with fluorine.

Physiology of chloramphenicol acetyltransferase synthesis

Chloramphenicol acetyltransferase, like β-lactamase, is an inducible enzyme in *S. aureus* but is constitutive in *E. coli*. It is remarkable that chloramphenicol, which is a potent inhibitor of protein biosynthesis, should promote the synthesis of the enzyme which destroys its inhibitory activity. Kinetic studies of the induction process in *S. aureus* show that in the early phase there is a conflict between the ability of chloramphenicol to induce the synthesis of chloramphenicol acetyltransferase and its ability to inhibit protein biosynthesis. Eventually, sufficient enzyme is produced to depress the concentration of chloramphenicol below that needed to inhibit protein synthesis. Since this concentration of antibiotic still effectively induces enzyme synthesis, the production of chloramphenicol acetyl transferase now proceeds rapidly.

An analogue of chloramphenicol, 3-deoxychloramphenicol, induces chloramphenicol acetyl transferase but does not inhibit protein bio-synthesis; it is not a substrate for chloramphenicol acetyl transferase. When 3-deoxychloramphenicol is used to induce chloramphenicol acetyltransferase the biosynthesis of the enzyme proceeds without the prolonged lag that is observed with chloramphenicol.

Comparison of chloramphenicol acetyltransferases from gram-positive and gram-negative cells

Preparations of chloramphenicol acetyltransferase isolated from extracts of *S. aureus* and R^+ *E.coli* have molecular weights of approximately 80 000; the pH optima are also similar (7 to 8). There are, however, significant differences in other properties:

(i)   The substrate affinity of the *S. aureus* enzyme is about 2.5 times greater than that of the *E.coli* enzyme.

(ii) While the *E.coli* enzyme is rapidly inactivated at 75°C, the *S. aureus* enzyme shows remarkable stability at this temperature.

(iii) There is no immunological cross-reactivity between the two enzymes.

(iv) While there is extensive amino acid sequence homology among the chloramphenicol acetyltransferases of Gram-negative bacteria, the sequences of transferases from Gram-positive bacteria are widely different. There is, however, sequence homology in the chloramphenicol-binding site regions of the *S. aureus* enzyme and those of Gram-negative bacteria enzymes.

There are differences among chloramphenicol acetyltransferases specified by different R-factors. In particular, the enzyme determined by fi⁻ R-factors, which only infrequently carry resistance to chloramphenicol, shows significant electrophoretic, immunological and catalytic differences from the enzyme coded by fi⁺ R-factors. Certain strains of *P. mirabilis* which are moderately resistant to chloramphenicol produce a chloramphenicol acetyltransferase that is chromosomally determined. The enzyme has a considerable resemblance to the chloramphenicol acetyltransferase coded by fi^+ R-factors and it has been inferred from this that the R-factor locus for the enzyme might have originated from a 'pick up' during a period of R-factor integration into the chromosome.

Inactivation of aminoglycoside antibiotics

The discovery of enzymes from aminoglycoside-resistant bacteria that convert the aminoglycosides to biologically inert products seemed at first to place aminoglycoside resistance in the same category as resistance to β-lactams and chloramphenicol. More extensive investigations have revealed, however, that the basic principle of aminoglycoside resistance may be subtly different. Enzymic modification of aminoglycosides, which occurs in the periplasmic space or on the cytoplasmic membrane, has a double effect. Firstly the modified compound is unable to induce the polyamine-transport system needed to permit rapid entry of unchanged drug into the cell, and secondly the inhibitory action on cell growth and division is lost because the modified compound no longer affects the ribosomal target.

The aminoglycosides, apart from certain common features, are molecularly remarkably varied. It is not surprising, therefore, that bacteria have evolved a range of defensive enzymes to deploy against them. Fortunately, however, the aminoglycosides undergo only three basic mechanisms of enzymic inactivation: (i) *phosphorylation,* (ii) *adenylation* and (iii) *acetylation.* Phosphorylation and adenylation occur at susceptible OH groups and acetylation at certain NH_2 groups. Enzymes carrying out these reactions have been detected in Gram-positive and Gram-negative bacteria. Some representative reactions are illustrated in Fig. 8.7

In Gram-negative bacteria the genes for the aminoglycoside-modifying enzymes are carried on R-factors and several of these genes are found on transposons. Plasmids also carry the enzyme genes in Gram-positive organisms. Usually, the synthesis of amino-glycoside-modifying enzymes is constitutive, although this aspect of aminoglycoside-resistance has not been studied in any detail. There is some evidence that several of the enzymes are subject to catabolite repression.

For a comprehensive account of the known aminoglycoside-modifying enzymes the reader should consult a recent review mentioned at the end of this chapter. In summary, the three mechanisms involving phosphorylation, adenylation and acetylation can be further subdivided according to the specific OH and NH_2 groups that are involved in the reaction. Thus there are five different types of *O*-phosphotransferases, four types of *O*-nucleotidyltransferases and three *N*-acetyltransferases. New enzymes are continually being discovered and more subgroups can be expected to appear within the basic mechanisms of aminoglycoside inactivation.

Phosphorylation of susceptible OH groups requires ATP as the phosphate donor, and the same nucleotide provides AMP for the adenylation reaction. Streptomycin is a substrate for both an *O*-phosphotransferase and an *O*-nucleotidyltransferase, the same OH being attacked by each (Fig. 8.7). The widespread *N*-acetylation reaction requires the transfer of an acetyl group from acetyl-CoA to an NH_2 group and it only affects those antibiotics with a deoxystrepamine moiety (Fig. 8.7); streptomycin and spectinomycin are

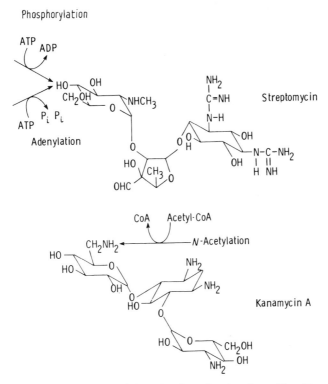

Figure 8.7 Three modes of enzymic inactivation of aminoglycosides. Streptomycin is not subject to *N*-acetylation, but kanamycin A is also inactivated by adenylation and phosphorylation.

thus immune from this type of inactivation. N-Acetylation is not invariably associated with cellular resistance. Tobramycin, for example, is a relatively poor substrate for the N-acetyltransferase that readily inactivates gentamicin C_{1a} (the 3-amino group of the deoxystrepamine ring is attacked). Bacteria that produce this enzyme are resistant to gentamicin C_{1a} but are quite sensitive to tobramycin. Presumably tobramycin is not N-acetylated quickly enough to limit its entry into the bacterial cells. Recent evidence suggests the emergence of a new form of this N-acetyltransferase which more effectively acetylates tobramycin and causes cellular resistance in pathogenic bacteria.

Since the aminoglycosides are subject to the development of resistance by more than one inactivation mechanism and by an extraordinary range of enzymes, strenuous efforts have been made to discover chemical modifications which might protect them from this enzymic onslaught. Amikacin, for example, is a synthetic derivative of kanamycin A with a hydroxyaminobutyric acid side chain substituted at the l-amino position. This substitution renders amikacin resistant to attack by all the aminoglycoside-modifying enzymes with the exception of kanamycin N-acetyl transferase and a recently discovered phosphotransferase specific for amikacin. The drug has been used successfully against infections caused by Gram-negative bacteria that are resistant to other aminoglycosides.

(2) Modification of the drug-sensitive site

Streptomycin

A striking example of the modification of a drug-sensitive site resulting in a high level of resistance is the loss of ribosomal sensitivity to streptomycin referred to in Chapter 5. The change in ribosomal structure has been traced to a single amino acid replacement in either of two positions in the S12 protein of the 30S ribosomal subunit. The changes in the S12 protein are caused by chromosomal mutations. The modified 30S subunit no longer binds streptomycin and the drug cannot therefore exert its characteristic effects on protein biosynthesis. The S12 protein may also be modified in mutants showing streptomycin-dependence. Streptomycin-resistance due to modified ribosomes is much less significant clinically than the plasmid-mediated resistance, although some clinical isolates of *Streptococcus faecalis* resistant to streptomycin have altered ribosomes with streptomycin-resistant 30S subunits.

Kasugamycin

This is an aminoglycoside antibiotic with an action on the 30S subunit of 70S ribosomes not unlike that of spectinomycin, i.e. it inhibits protein synthesis but it does not induce misreading nor can it cause phenotypic suppression. Kasugamycin-resistant mutants can be isolated with resistant 30S subunits that are unusual in having altered ribosomal RNA instead of protein. The mutation causes a loss in the activity of an enzyme that specifically methylates two adenine residues to dimethyl adenine in the sequence, A-A-C-C-U-G, near the 3' end of the 16S RNA. It is assumed that the change in the 16S RNA hinders the normal interaction between kasugamycin and the ribosome, but, owing to the weak binding of the drug to sensitive ribosomes, it has not been possible to demonstrate unequivocally that there is diminished binding to resistant ribosomes. It is interesting to find that 30S subunits from kasugamycin-resistant cells are methylated by the methylase from sensitive cells. When these methylated subunits are recombined with 50S subunits the resultant 70S particles are sensitive to kasugamycin.

Erythromycin

Resistance to this drug in several bacterial species depends on an alteration in a protein of the 50S subunit. The protein involved may be either L4 or L12; in either event the change leads to a reduced affinity of the ribosome for erythromycin. In *S. aureus*, however, the 23S RNA of the 50S subunit is modified. An inducible, plasmid-mediated ribosomal RNA methylase is responsible for the alteration in the 23S RNA which involves dimethylation of a specific adenine moiety. The modified ribosomes are cross-resistant to lincomycin. This mechanism of resistance provides an intriguing contrast with that of kasugamycin where a specific loss of RNA methylation is involved.

Rifamycins

Another important example of a mutation causing a change in the drug-sensitive site is seen in the altered DNA-dependent RNA polymerase found in mutants resistant to the rifamycin antibiotics. As we saw in Chapter 4, resistance to the rifamycins depends on a modification of the β-subunit of the 'core' enzyme of the polymerase. Loss of sensitivity of the polymerase to rifampicin is accompanied by a failure of the 'core' enzyme to bind the antibiotic. The change in the enzyme is determined by a chromosomal mutation.

It is not possible for an organism to acquire resistance to every inhibitor by modification of the appropriate target site. Some changes that would confer resistance are almost certainly incompatible with cell viability. The consistent failure to isolate bacterial mutants with tetracycline-resistant ribosomes, for example, could be explained if such resistant ribosomes were non-functional in protein biosynthesis.

(3) Loss of cell permeability to a drug

Several mechanisms of resistance mimic a fall in cell permeability to a drug. A familiar example is where resistant cells convert a drug to a derivative that does not bind to its intracellular target. The cells no longer sequester the drug and a false impression of changed permeability is created. Similarly, a change in the target site leading to a loss of affinity for a drug results in a diminished cellular uptake of drug. The conversion of aminoglycoside antibiotics to derivatives that cannot induce the active uptake of aminoglycosides provides another example of an apparent change in cellular permeability to the parent molecules.

Despite these traps for the unwary, resistance to certain anti-microbial drugs clearly depends on cellular changes that hinder drug access. This loss of permeability may be due to one of several mechanisms:

(i)   An additional permeability barrier may be synthesized. The greater intrinsic antibiotic insensitivity of Gram-negative bacteria compared with Gram-positive organisms depends on the non-specific permeability barrier provided by the outer membrane of Gram-negative cells (Chapter 7). Mutants of *S. typhimurium* and *E.coli* are known that have an enhanced resistance to ampicillin that appears to be associated with specific changes in the polysaccharide components of the cell envelopes. In these cases it seems that the nature of the permeability barrier is modified so as to reduce the rate of movement of antibiotic through it. The reduced uptake of streptomycin and erythromycin by some resistant pneumococci may be explained by the development of a permeability barrier. Since these resistant strains are less susceptible to DNA transformation because of a diminished uptake of transforming DNA, the permeability barrier is probably non-specific.

(ii)   When the antimicrobial substance gains intracellular access by a specific transport mechanism, diminished uptake of the drug by resistant cells can be due to a mutation that affects some component of the permeation mechanism resulting in a partial or complete loss of transport function. A drug resembling a natural nutrient can be transported into cells by a permeation mechanism designed for the nutrient. If the permeation mechanism fails in some cells the resistant cell population may emerge. A good example of this mechanism is found in a series of mutants of *E.coli* resistant to D-cycloserine. In sensitive cells this drug is accumulated by the amino acid-transport system that normally carries D-alanine or glycine. Mutants exhibit a graded loss of function of this transport system which is associated with a progressive increase in resistance to cycloserine.

In Gram-negative bacteria the contribution of the pore and solute receptor proteins of the outer membrane to drug penetration should also be remembered (Chapter 7). A mutant of *E.coli* that lacks two pore proteins is unable to take up several low-molecular-weight solutes including chloramphenicol, thus making the mutant resistant to this antibiotic. This type of resistance is, however, very much a product of the research laboratory and is not clinically significant.

(iii) Specific antagonism of antibiotic transport. The most commonly encountered mode of resistance to tetracyclines in Gram-positive and Gram-negative bacteria, which is of considerable medical importance, depends on diminished cellular permeability to the drugs. Many tetracycline-sensitive bacteria accumulate tetracyclines by an energy-dependent process which involves the cytoplasmic membrane (Chapter 7). Tetracycline transport in resistant cells is blocked by a partially inducible system that is determined by extra-chromosomal genes in Gram-positive and Gram-negative bacteria. Tetracycline-resistant cells typically exhibit two levels of resistance. The sensitivity of protein biosynthesis to tetracycline in R^+ *E.coli* is about 50-100 times less at bacteriostatic concentrations than in sensitive R^- cells. At higher concentrations of tetracycline there is increasing inhibition of the R^+ cells. There is a clear indication that R^+ cells accumulate less tetracycline than do R^- cells. When the resistant cells are exposed to a subinhibitory concentration of tetracycline there is a further rapid increase in the level of resistance which can be prevented by blocking protein or RNA synthesis in the cells. The increase in resistance is associated with a further fall in the uptake of tetracycline by the cells. A similar process occurs in *S. aureus* resistant to tetracycline. There is no evidence that the antibiotic is chemically modified by the resistant cells.

In R-factor-mediated tetracycline-resistance in *E.coli* at least three proteins are induced by the tetracyclines. These proteins appear to be located in the cell envelope, although one protein with a molecular weight of 15 000 may occur in both the cytoplasm and the cytoplasmic membrane. The other proteins are associated with the outer envelope of the bacterial cell. At present the contribution of these proteins to cellular resistance to tetracyclines is unknown. In Gram-negative bacteria hydrophilic tetracyclines traverse the outer membrane via the pore proteins. Resistance proteins associated with the outer envelope might therefore hinder the movement of tetracyclines through the pores. Another suggestion is that one protein may bind to the ribosomes and interfere with the inhibition of protein synthesis by tetracyclines. Finally it even is possible that tetracyclines are pumped out of resistant cells as soon as they enter. It will be realized, therefore, that the mechanism of resistance to the tetracyclines is proving exceptionally difficult to unravel.

The genes that determine tetracycline resistance in Gram-negative bacteria are frequently found on transposon 10, although the genes may not be contiguous with each other. Transposon 10 is a component of several R-factors. However, there are other phenotypically similar determinants of tetracycline-resistance that may be only distantly related to that on transposon 10 or may even have evolved independently of it. In *S. aureus* the determinant for tetracycline-resistance frequently occurs on plasmids that are between 2.7 and 2.8 megadaltons. The widespread occurrence of tetracycline-resistance among staphylococci may well be due to the plasmid location of the resistance genes and the possible involvement of a transposon.

(4) Provision of an alternative enzyme or pathway that bypasses the inhibited reaction

Resistance to the sulphonamides has been recognized for nearly forty years and the resistance determinant was found on R-factors when they were first discovered in Japan in the 1950s. However, only in the last few years has the mechanism of R-factor-mediated resistance to sulphonamides been revealed. The plasmid carries the genetic information for a form of dihydropteroate synthetase that is highly resistant to inhibition by the sulphonamides. The chromosomally determined form of this enzyme (Chapter 6) is the target of the sulphonamides. R-factor-determined dihydropteroate synthetase is 1000 times less sensitive to sulphathiazole than the chromosomal enzyme, while the K_m for the substrate, *p*-aminobenzoic acid, is the same for both enzymes. Cells with the R-factor-determined enzyme utilize *p*-aminobenzoic acid normally, despite high concentrations of sulphonamides. Pneumococci resistant to sulphonamides synthesize a similar dihydropteroate synthetase that is not inhibited by sulphonamides.

The sulphonamide, sulphamethoxazole, is often used in

combination with trimethoprim (Chapter 6). It was believed that resistance to this combination would be slow to emege. However, bacteria causing serious infections are now appearing that harbour R-factors with resistance markers for both sulphonamides and trimethoprim. The mechanism of trimethoprim-resistance follows the same principle as sulphonamide-resistance; the plasmid carries a gene that directs the synthesis of a dihydrofolate reductase which is highly resistant to trimethoprim. The K_m for the substrate, dihydrofolate, is similar to that of the chromosomally determined trimethoprim-sensitive enzyme. In fact there are two forms of trimethoprim-resistant enzymes determined by R-factors. Type I enzymes are several thousand times more resistant to trimethoprim than the chromosomal enzyme, whilst Type II enzymes are almost totally resistant to trimethoprim. Interestingly, both types of enzyme are highly resistant to methotrexate which is a close structural analogue of dihydrofolate. Recently a Type II enzyme from *E. coli* has been extensively characterized. In contrast with the monomeric chromosomal enzyme that has a molecular weight of 18 000, the Type II enzyme is a tetramer with a total molecular weight of 34 000.

Resistance to a metabolic inhibitor is also possible if alternative or bypass reactions or routes are enhanced. Examples of possible bypass reactions are found in the pathways of purine and pyrimidine nucleotide metabolism. These are known as the salvage pathways, since purine and pyrimidine bases or their nucleosides arising from catabolic processes are converted to the corresponding nucleotides and reutilized for nucleic acid biosynthesis or nucleotide cofactor function. Clearly, these salvage reactions provide the means of escape from nucleotide deprivation caused by inhibitors of biosynthesis of purine and pyrimidine nucleotides *de novo*. Sensitivity and resistance of tumour cells to inhibitors of the purine and pyrimidine nucleotide pathways may be determined by these salvage pathways. The activities of the enzymes that catalyse the salvage reactions (purine and pyrimidine phosphoribosyl transferases and nucleoside phosphorylases) vary widely in both normal and malignant mammalian tissues. Although the factors controlling these variations are unknown, this flexibility furnishes a means of circumventing the inhibition of synthesis *de novo*, provided that adequate supplies of exogenous purine and pyrimidine bases or their nucleosides are available. While similar bypass mechanisms could account for resistance to inhibitors of purine and pyrimidine biosynthesis in microbial cells, this mechanism does not appear to be of significance in resistance to the clinically important antimicrobial drugs affecting nucleotide biosynthesis.

(5) Increased production of a drug-sensitive enzyme

If an organism can achieve a substantially increased synthesis of a target enzyme, it stands a chance of overcoming the inhibition by a drug of the formation of the product of the enzyme reaction. Increased synthesis of a repressible enzyme can result from mutations affecting the repressor itself or the operator gene with which the repressor interacts. An interesting example of microbial resistance that depends on a loss of repressor control over inducible enzymes is seen in bacterial mutants resistant to the amino acid analogue 5-methyl tryptophan. The enzymes of the tryptophan biosynthetic pathway are normally co-ordinately repressed by tryptophan itself, since the repressor acts on an operator which controls the biosynthesis of all the enzymes in this pathway. In the mutants resistant to 5-methyltryptophan, tryptophan no longer exerts this control; the enzymes are fully induced at all times and excess tryptophan is biosynthesized. The immediate cause of resistance appears to be excess production of anthranilate synthetase, the enzyme inhibited by 5-methyltryptophan.

A class of mutants resistant to the purine nucleoside antibiotic psicofuranine produces a defective form of the enzyme IMP dehydrogenase (Chapter 4) that is unable to maintain a normal supply of XMP; the level of intracellular GMP is thus depressed. The biosynthesis of XMP aminase, which is the target enzyme of psicofuranine, is repressed by its end product GMP, and the diminished concentration of GMP in the mutant cells leads to extra production of XMP aminase. By elevating the concentration of the target enzyme in this way the cells escape from the growth-inhibiting effects of psicofuranine. The control of the rate of synthesis of constitutive enzymes is less well understood but examples are known where the synthesis of constitutive target enzymes is greatly enhanced in resistant cells. Resistance to amethopterin, an inhibitor of dihydrofolate reductase, depends in some mutants of *Lactobacillus casei* on greatly increased levels of the target enzyme. The amount of dihydrofolate reductase in resistant cells may be several-hundredfold greater than in sensitive bacteria.

At the present time resistance due to enhanced levels of target enzymes is confined to resistant mutants discovered in the laboratory and is probably of minimal clinical significance.

(6) Increased production of a metabolite that antagonizes the inhibitor

When an antimicrobial compound inhibits growth by the competitive antagonism of a normal metabolite, resistance to such an inhibitor may be due to increased production of the metabolite; the inhibitor is competitively displaced from its enzyme binding site. Among examples of this type of resistance are certain mutants resistant to sulphonamides. In these cells the concentration of p-aminobenzoic acid is said to be substantially higher than in sulphonamide-sensitive cells. Unfortunately, the mechanism underlying the increased production of p-aminobenzoic acid has never been explained. This mechanism of sulphonamide-resistance is probably much less important than that due to resistant dihydropteroate synthetase.

(7) Decreased requirement for the product of an inhibited reaction

This type of resistance is another version of the 'alternative route' mechanism. Thus while an inhibitor may block a step in a bio-synthetic sequence and cut off the supply of an essential end product, resistance can be achieved by using another route to the end product.

Organisms isolated from patients treated with the sulphamethoxazole-trimethoprim sometimes have a requirement for thymine or thymidine. Since the drug combination interferes with the normal supply of thymine compounds required for DNA synthesis, cellular resistance could occur if the bacteria acquired the necessary compounds from exogenous sources. This mechanism of resistance to sulphamethoxazole-trimethoprim is likely to be only of minor importance.

Practical approaches to the control of drug-resistance

We have reviewed the genetic and biochemical ingenuity of micro-organisms in combating the toxic effects of growth-inhibiting substances. Highly successful mechanisms of resistance against antibiotics were probably evolved by micro-organisms long before the introduction of these substances into medical and veterinary practice. The development of resistance against novel, chemically synthesized agents not resembling natural metabolites or growth factors is more difficult to explain, although the high rate of cell division in most microbial populations obviously facilitates 'high speed' evolution. Bacteria may acquire the genes for exotic, inhibitor-resistant enzymes from viral sources. While the occurrence of such resistant enzymes is fortuitous, the facile movement of genetic material in micro-organisms enables bacteria to exploit such opportunities for survival in the face of the antibacterial threat. Nevertheless, bacteria may possess only a limited capacity for developing effective resistance without sacrificing viability. Clinical experience with β-lactamase-stable penicillin derivatives such as methicillin gives some support to this view, since resistance to these derivatives has appeared much more slowly than to the original penicillin. It is also of interest that streptococci apparently do not become resistant to β-lactam antibiotics under practical conditions of use. A detailed consideration of the common mechanisms of resistance and their frequency of occurrence among important pathogens assists the design of new chemotherapeutic agents to which micro-organisms could adapt only with much greater difficulty. At the present time considerable efforts are being directed to the development of new β-lactams with improved stability to the many different bacterial β-lactamases.

Apart from the preparation of new chemical agents to combat drug-resistance, there are a number of other measures which can be taken:

(1) Treatment of an infection is usually begun with the administration of a high 'loading' dose of antimicrobial drug in the hope of suppressing the growth of any partially resistant organisms in the body. Therapy is continued with doses large enough and frequent enough to maintain an effective antibacterial level of drug in the blood until the infection is overcome.

(2) Micro-organisms are often cross-resistant to chemically related drugs. Simultaneous therapy with chemically unrelated inhibitors, however, presents a much more formidable challenge to a micro-organism especially when the inhibitors attack an essential metabolic route at two different points. Although R-factors conferring resistance to the sulphamethoxazole-trimethoprim combination are now appearing, several years of 'grace' were obtained before this occurred. In the treatment of tuberculosis, where the need for therapy extending over many months encourages the development of drug-resistance, the use of a combination of isoniazid, streptomycin and *p*-aminosalicylic acid successfully avoids the frequent emergence of resistant strains. The use in clinical medicine of combinations of inhibitors of β-lactamase and β-lactams could prove to be a useful approach to counter the threat of β-lactamase-producing pathogens.

(3) Undoubtedly, the careless use of antimicrobial agents in human medicine and in farming practice for non-therapeutic purposes has assisted the spread of resistant organisms. A recent

encouraging development, however, is towards insistence on much stricter control over the use of these drugs. The proper and careful deployment of antimicrobial agents can produce dramatic results in reducing the number of resistant organisms in the environment.

Further reading

General
J.D. WATSON (1977), *Molecular Biology of the Gene*, 3rd edn. (W.A. Benjamin Inc., 1977).
M.H. RICHMOND (1973), 'Resistance factors and their ecological importance to bacteria and man', in *Prog. Nucleic Acid Res. Mol. Biol.*, 13, 191.
R.W. LACEY (1973), 'Genetic basis, epidemiology and future significance of antibiotic resistance in *Staphylococcus aureus:* A review', in *J. Clin. Pathol.*, 26, 899.
M.R.W. BROWN (ed) (1975), *Resistance of Pseudomonas aeruginosa* (John Wiley & Sons, 1975).

Molecular genetics
D.R. HELINSKI (1973), 'Plasmid-determined resistance to antibiotics: Molecular properties of R-factors', in *Annu. Rev. Microbiol.*, 87, 473.
G.S. STENT and R. CALENDAR (1978), *Molecular Genetics, An Introductory Narrative*, 2nd edn. (W.H. Freeman and Company, 1978).
S.N. COHEN (1976), 'Transposable genetic elements and plasmid evolution', in *Nature (London)*, 263, 731.

Biochemical mechanisms of resistance
J. DAVIES and D.I. SMITH (1978), 'Plasmid-determined resistance to antimicrobial agents', in *Annu. Rev. Microbiol.*, 32, 469.
J.M.T. HAMILTON-SMITH and J.T. SMITH (eds) (1979), *Beta-lactamases* (Academic Press, 1979).
I. CHOPRA and T.G.B. HOWE (1978), 'Bacterial resistance to the tetracyclines', in *Microbiol. Rev.*, 42, 707.
F.E. HAHN (1980) 'New derivatives of chloramphenicol active against resistant bacteria', in *Naturwissenschaften*, 67, 89.
D. STONE and S.L. SMITH (1979), 'The amino acid sequence of the trimetho-prim-resistant dihydrofolate reductase specified in *Escherichia coli* by R-plasmid R67', in *J. Biol. Chem.*, 254, 10851.

Index

A23187
  causes release of Mg from
  mitochondria, 72
  ionophor specific for divalent ions, 72
  preferential binding of Ca, 72
  structure, 71
Acceptor in peptidoglycan biosynthesis,
  31, 33
Acceptor site, in protein biosynthesis,
  112, 114
Acetylation
  of aminoglycosides, 192, 193, 194
  of chloramphenicol, 189, 190, 191,
  192
Acridines, 88
  binding to DNA, 89
  inhibition of nucleic acid synthesis
  by, 89, 95
  medical history, 88
  vital staining, 89
Acriflavine, 4
Actinomycin D,
  discovery, 89
  inhibition of RNA synthesis by, 95
  interaction with DNA, 90, 91, 92
  structural features, 89, 90
  uses, 90
Activation of amino acids, 111
  inhibition by amino acid analogues
  and antibiotics, 117, 118
Activation of antimicrobial compounds
  by metabolism, 7, 8
Active transport of antimicrobial
  agents, 162
Acyclovir
  antiviral, 156
  structure, 157
Adenosine, resemblance to psicofuranine,
  83
Adenosine triphosphatase from
  mitochondria, structure, 148
Adenosine triphosphatase, inhibition
  by A23187, 72
  inhibition by oligomycin, 148
  in membrane, inhibition by
  chlorhexidine, 62
Adenosine triphosphate, interference
  by antimicrobial agents, 8
Adenylation of aminoglycosides, 192, 193
Adenylosuccinate synthetase, 83

Adenylosuccinic acid, 83
Affinity for drugs, diminished in
  resistance, 8, 194, 195, 196
Alaphosphin
  action, 170
  structure, 169
  uptake by bacteria, 169, 170
D-Alanine
  antagonism of antibacterial action
  of cycloserine, 40
  liberation in cross-linking of
  peptidoglycan, 33
  release in peptidoglycan cross-linking
  inhibited by penicillin, 48
D-Alanine carboxypeptidases
  in bacterial wall, 36
  in membrane preparations, 49
  inhibition by penicillin, 49
Alanine permeases, in accumulation of
  D-cycloserine, 166
Alanine racemase, 30
  inhibition by alaphosphin, 170
  inhibition by cycloserine, 40
D-Alanyl-D-alanine end group, structural
  resemblance to penicillin, 51
D-Alanyl-D-alanine synthetase, 30
  inhibition by cycloserine, 40
  in peptidoglycan biosynthesis, 30
Allosteric sites, alteration during
  enzyme purification, 17
Amantadine
  biochemical action, 157
  prophylaxis against influenza A_2, 157
  structure, 157
Amikacin, resistance to aminoglycoside
  modifying enzymes, 194
Amino acids, leakage from Gram-positive
  bacteria caused by antiseptics, 60
p-Aminobenzoic acid
  as a bacterial growth factor, 140
  competitive antagonism of
  sulphonamide action, 140
  isostere of sulphonamides, 140
  part of the structure of folic acid, 140
7-Aminocephalosporanic acid, 44, 45
Aminoglycoside antibiotics
  acetylation, 192, 193, 194
  action on protein synthesis, 121, 122
  adenylation, 192, 193
  killing action of, 133

resistance, 120, 192, 193, 194
phosphorylation, 192, 193, 194
uptake by bacteria, 168
(*see also* Amikacin, Streptomycin,
Neomycin, Kanamycin, Gentamicin,
Spectinomycin)
6-Aminopenicillanic acid, 44, 45
p-Aminosalicylic acid, use in tuberculosis,
139
Amoebic dysentery, treatment with
emetine, 3
Amoxycillin, 44, 45
Amphotericin B, 75
synergism with other antifungal
agents, 170, 171
Ampicillin, 44, 45
binding to proteins 2 and 3 of
cytoplasmic membrane, 53
Amprolium, inhibition of thiamine
uptake, 155
structure, 156
4*a*, 12*a*-Anhydro tetracycline, 125
Antibacterial action, information from
auxotrophic bacteria, 15
reversal by biologically important
compounds, 15
Antibacterials for systemic use,
bacteriostasis is sufficient, 58
Antibiotics
discovery, 11
forming complexes with potassium, 69
the heyday of their development, 11
selective biochemical actions, 12
semi-synthetic, 12
Anticancer drugs, 79, 80, 81, 82, 84,
90, 92, 94, 95, 107
Antigenic groups in Gram-negative wall,
26
Antifungal agents, 151
Antimicrobial action
comparison of effects *in vivo* and
in vitro, 16
evidence from effect on uptake of
nutrients, 16
relationship to chemical structure, 18
selectivity towards micro-organisms, 17
Antimicrobial agents
distinction between primary and
secondary effects, 14
early remedies, 2
metabolism in the body, 13
necessary biological features, 18
pharmacological biochemistry, 13
protein binding, 13
selectivity through concentration in
the microbial cell, 17
social and economic importance, 1
structural analogies with biologically
important molecules, 15
Antimonials, preferential inhibition of
phosphofructokinase of schistosomes,
154
Antimycin
action on fungi, yeasts and subcellular

particles, 145
as fish poison, 147
lack of action on bacteria or bacterial
enzymes, 145
point of action in the cytochrome
system, 146
Antimycin A$_1$, structure, 146
Antiprotozoal drugs, 89, 154
Antisepsis, early attempts, 3
Antiseptics, 58
bacteriostatic action at low
concentration, 59
causing leakage of cytoplasmic
constituents, 60
early history, 3
factors in bactericidal action, 59
need for bactericidal action, 59
penetration into bacterial cells, 60, 64
uptake by bacterial cytoplasmic
membrane, 61
Ara A, *see* Arabinosyl adenine
Arabinogalactan, in walls of
mycobacteria, 37
Arabinosyl adenine
inhibition of DNA synthesis, 107, 108
structure, 106
uses, 107
Arabinosyl cytosine
inhibition of DNA synthesis, 107,
108
structure, 106
uses, 107
Ara C, *see* Arabinosyl cytosine
Arsenicals
binding to lipoic acid, 154
inhibition of oxidative decarboxylation of *a*-keto acids, 154
separation of toxicity and
chemotherapeutic activity, 5
suggested mode of action, 14
Arsenious oxide, as trypanocide, 5
Asepsis, 4
L-Aspartic acid, analogue, 82, 83
Atebrin, *see* Mepacrine
Atoxyl
resistance in trypanosomes, 8
structure, 6
Auxotrophic bacteria, use in determining
site of antibacterial action, 15
Azaserine
clinical use, 81
inhibition of purine nucleotide
synthesis, 81, 82
radiomimetic and mutagenic
properties, 82
structure, 82

Bacitracin, binding to pyrophosphates, 53
complex formation with undecaprenyl
pyrophosphate, 54
complex formation with farnesyl
pyrophosphate, 54
structure, 55
uses and antibacterial action, 53

Bacteria, uncertainty of death, 59
Bacterial cell, differences from animal
    cells, 21
Bacterial cell wall
    permeability function, 162, 163, 164
    protective function, 21
Bacteriophage, *see* Phage
Bacteriostatic and bactericidal action
    compared, 59
Bacteriostatic drugs, in the treatment
    of systemic infections, 7
Benomyl
    agricultural fungicide, 153
    effect on chromosome separation, 153
    metabolism to MBC, 153
    structure, 153
Benzyl penicillin, 43, 44
    affinity for β-lactamase, 187
Biocides, 58
Biosynthetic pathways, methods of
    determining sites of blockage, 15
Bleomycin A, structure, 94
Bleomycins, action of DNA, 94, 95
Bone marrow, toxic effects of
    chloramphenicol on, 135, 136
Borrelidin, 117
Bridging groups, variation in different
    types of peptidoglycan, 35
Broad spectrum antibiotics, definition,
    118
Buquinolate, 155, 156

Calcium
    binding to A23187, 72
    significance in Gram-negative bacterial
    wall, 26, 163
Candida albicans infections, treated with
    miconazole, 152
Carbenicillin, 44, 45
Carbodox, 149
Carboxin
    agricultural fungicide, 147
    blocks succinate branch of respiratory
    pathway, 147
DD-Carboxypeptidase I, 36
Carboxypeptidase II, 36
Carboxypeptidase action, compared with
    transpeptidase action, 49
Carboxypeptidases
    active centre, 50
    extracellular, from streptomycetes, 49
    reaction intermediates, 50
    with transpeptidase activity, 49
Cationic antiseptics, 61
Cefoxitin, 44, 46
    stability to β-lactamase, 188
Cefuroxime, 44, 46
    stability to β-lactamase, 188
Cell envelope, 21
Cephalexin, 44, 46
    binding to protein 3 of cytoplasmic
    membrane, 53
Cephalosporanic acid, instability, 185
Cephaloridine, 44, 46

Cephalosporin C, 44, 45
Cephalosporins and penicillins
    biosynthesis, 45
    semi-synthetic, 45
    structure, 44
Cephalothin, 44
Cephamycin C, 44, 46
Cerulenin
    action antagonized by fatty acids, 56
    structure and action, 55
Cetrimide
    causes leakage of P from *E. coli,* 62
    chain length and antiseptic action, 62
    structure, 61
Chain, Ernst Boris, 11
Chelation of cations by tetracyclines, 126
Chemical structure, related to
    antimicrobial action, 18
Chemotherapy
    early history, 4
    its debt to Ehrlich, 6
Chitin biosynthesis, inhibition by
    polyoxins, 56
Chloramphenicol
    binding to ribosomes, 126, 127
    clinical use, 126
    derivatives resistant to chloram-
    phenicol acetyltransferase, 191
    effect on bone marrow, 135, 136
    effect on yeast cells, 135
    inhibition of peptide bond formation,
    128
    inhibition of puromycin reaction, 128
    manufacture, 126
    resistance, 189 ff.
    side effects, 126, 135, 136
    specificity of action, 126
    structure, 127
    uptake by bacterial cells, 164, 165
Chloramphenicol acetyltransferase
    action of, 189, 190
    comparison in Gram-positive and
    Gram-negative organisms, 191, 192
    synthesis, 190, 191
Chloramphenicol acetylase, *see*
    Chloramphenicol acetyltransferase
Chlorhexidine
    antagonism of membrane adenosine
    triphosphatase, 62
    'blistering' of cell wall, 64
    leakage of bacterial cytoplasmic
    components diminished at high
    concentrations, 64
    low concentrations inhibit bacterial
    uptake of potassium, 62
    physical and antiseptic properties, 62
    possible use in trachoma, 62
    precipitation of bacterial nucleic
    acid and protein, 64
    slow release from tissues, 62
    structure, 61
    use in dental hygiene, 62
Chloride of lime, as disinfectant, 3
Chloroplasts, 70S ribosomes, 111, 135

Chloroquine
    interaction with DNA, 89
    structure, 88
Chlortetracycline, 123
Chromosomes, drug resistance genes, 174, 176, 178, 179
Cinchona bark, 2
Clavulanic acid
    inhibitor of β-lactamase, 47, 188
    structure, 46
Clindamycin
    action on ribosomes, 130
    structure, 130
Clostridial infections of the gut, treated with vancomycin, 42
Cloxacillin, 44, 45
Coccidiosis, occurrence and treatment in chicks, 155
Codon misreadings, induction of by aminoglycosides, 119, 121
Concentration of antimicrobial agents in microbial cells, 17, 159
Conjugation
    bacterial, physiology of, 181, 182, 183
    transfer of drug-resistance by, 177, 178, 179, 180, 181, 182, 183
Core enzyme, of RNA polymerase, 100, 101
Cotrimoxazole, 144
    double block in tetrahydrofolate biosynthesis, 145
Cross-linking to existing peptides in the wall, 33
Cycloheximide
    action on ribosomes, 132
    action on translocation, 132
    antimicrobial action, 132
    inhibition of translocation, 132
    resistance to, 132
    structure, 132
Cycloserine
    active uptake by bacteria, 40, 166
    antagonism of antibacterial effect by D-alanine, 40
    inhibition of alanine racemase and D-alanyl-D-alanine synthetase, 40
    mechanism of bacterial resistance, 197
    significance of rigid structure, 40
    structure and use, 39
Cyclosporin A
    immunosuppressive agent, 67
    structure, 68
Cytochrome *b*, site of action of antimycin, 147
Cytoplasmic constituents, leakage caused by antiseptics, 60
Cytoplasmic membrane,
    binding of polymyxin, 66
    as a permeability barrier to anti-microbial agents, 159
    site of absorption of antiseptics, 61

Dapsone, *see* 4, 4'-Diaminodiphenyl sulphone
Decoyinine, 83, 84
3, 4-Dehydroproline, 117
3-Deoxy-D-*manno*-octulosonic acid
    binding of Ca^{2+} and Mg^{2+}, 26
    component of lipopolysaccharide core, 26, 27
Deoxyribose, importance in DNA-actinomycin D interaction, 90
Depsipeptide antibiotics, 68
4, 4'-Diaminodiphenyl sulphone, use in leprosy, 139
Diaminopimelic acid, in peptidoglycan, 35
2, 6-Diaminopurine, in synthetic DNA polymers, 90
2, 4-Diaminopyrimidine, structural feature of dihydrofolate reductase inhibitors, 143
6-Diazo-5-oxo-L-norleucine
    action on purine nucleotide synthesis, 81, 82
    structure, 82
Diclobutrazole
    inhibition of sterol biosynthesis, 152
    structure, 153
Diffusion, 159
    facilitated, 161, 162, 166, 167, 168, 169
    passive, 160, 161, 165, 166
Dihydrofolate reductase
    differences between bacterial and mammalian enzyme, 144
    trimethoprim-resistant forms, 199
Dihydrofolate reductase inhibitors
    resistance to, 199
    specificity towards different organisms, 144
Dihydropteroate synthetase, sulphonamide-resistant form, 198
Dihydropteroic acid, biosynthesis inhibited *in vitro* by sulphonamides, 140
Disaccharide decapeptide, 31
Disinfectant, use of proflavine, 88
Disinfectants, 58
    chemically reactive, 59
    early history, 3
    modern uses, 4
    need for bactericidal action, 59
Dithiocarbamates, as fungicides, 151
DNA
    cross-linking by drugs, 95, 96, 97
    degradation by bleomycins, 94, 95
    degradation in mitomycin-treated cells, 97
    effects of actinomycin D on physical properties, 90, 92
    effects of intercalating drugs on physical properties, 86, 87
    gyrase, 105
    interaction with actinomycin D, 89, 90, 91, 92

interaction with quinoxaline antibiotics, 92, 93
local unwinding to allow intercalation, 86
polymerases, 102
swivelase, 104, 105
DNA synthesis inhibition
by actinomycin D, 95
by arabinosyl adenine, 107, 108
by arabinosyl cytosine, 107, 108
by hydroxphenylazopyrimidines, 102, 103, 104
by inhibitors of protein synthesis, 134, 135
by intercalating dyes, 95
by mitomycins, 97
by nalidixic acid, 104, 105
by novobiocin, 105
by oxolinic acid, 105
DNA circular, interaction with intercalating molecules, 87, 88
Domagk, Gerhardt, 9
DON, *see* 6-Diazo-5-oxo-L-norleucine
Donor site, in protein biosynthesis, 112, 114
Doxycycline, structure, 123
Drug-resistance, 172 ff.

Echinomycin
interaction with DNA, 92, 93
structure, 92, 93
Ehrlich, Paul, 5, 6, 9, 14
Emetine, 2
Enduracidin A
properties and action, 41
structure, 41
4-Epitetracycline, 125
Erythromycin
antibacterial action, 128
binding to ribosomes, 128, 129
effect of pH on antibacterial activity of, 161
effect on yeast cells, 135
effect on *Chlamydomonas,* 135
effect on *Euglena,* 135
inhibition of translocation, 129
site of ribosomal resistance to, 195
structure, 129
Ethanolamine, component of lipopolysaccharide core, 26, 27
Ethidium,
action on trypanosomal DNA, 88
action on yeast mitochondria, 88
structure, 88
Ethionine, 117
Ethylenediaminetetraacetic acid
disruption of Gram-negative outer envelope, 163
enhancement of permeability of Gram-negative bacteria, 163
Ethylene oxide, 59
N-Ethylglycine, 117
Eukaryotic cells, effects of inhibitors of protein synthesis on, 135, 136

Facilitated diffusion, 161, 162
of antimicrobial agents, 162, 166, 167, 168, 169
Ferrimycin A_1, 151
Ferrioxamine B, 151
FGAR, *see* Formyglycineamide ribonucleotide
Filamentous forms of *E. coli,* following treatment with β-lactams, 53
Fleming, Alexander, 10
Florey, Howard Walter, 11
Folic acid analogues
impermeability to bacterial cells, 142
toxicity, 142
N-Formyl hydroxyaminoacetic acid, *see* Hadacidin
N-Formyl methionine, 133
N-Formyl methionyl tRNA$_F$ role in protein biosynthesis, 133
Formylglycineamide ribonucleotide, accumulation of, 81
Fungal hyphae, affected by griseofulvin, 152
Fungal infections, treatment with nystatin, 75
Fungicides, 151
advantage of systemic use in plants, 152
affecting sterol biosynthesis, 152
Furanomycin, 117
Fusidic acid
clinical use, 131
inhibition of translocation, 131
resistance to, 131
structure, 131

Gentamicin
biochemical action, 121, 122
resistance, 194
structure, 122
Glutamine, analogues, 80, 81, 82
L-α-Glycerophosphate permease, transport of phosphomycin, 168
Glycine-specific transfer RNA, in peptidoglycan biosynthesis, 31
Glycopeptide, *see* Peptidoglycan
Gram-negative bacteria
intrinsic resistance to certain antibacterial agents, 162, 163, 164
synthetic capabilities, 22
Gram-negative bacterial walls, 24
chemical composition, 25
electron microscopy, 24
linkage of lipoprotein and peptidoglycan, 27, 37
role in resistance to antibacterial agents, 163, 164
structure, 26
Gram-positive bacteria
nutritional needs, 22
osmotic pressure, 22
Gram-positive bacterial walls, 22
Gramicidin A
biochemical action, 74
effect on membrane conductivity, 74

pore formation in membranes, 74
structure, 73
Gramicidin S, 64, 65, 66
    activity of analogues, 67
    conformation in solution, 67
    structural requirements for activity, 67
Griseofulvin, 152
    selective inhibition of fungal
    microtubule formation, 153
    structure, 153
GTP, role in protein biosynthesis, 113,
    114, 115
Guanine, importance in DNA-actinomycin
    D interaction, 90, 91
Guanine nucleotides, inhibition of
    biosynthesis by mycophenolic acid, 85
Guanosine, 84

Hadacidin
    clinical use, 82
    inhibition of purine nucleotide
    synthesis by, 83
    structure, 82
Halogens, 59
Halophilic bacteria, resistance to
    antibiotics affecting peptidoglycan
    synthesis, 38
Hansch equation, application to anti-
    bacterial agents, 160
Haptophore, 7
Herpes, treated with 5-iododeoxyuridine,
    106, 156
Hexachlorophene
    action and uses, 61
    effect on bacterial permeability, 61
    structure, 61
Hexose-6-phosphate permeases, in
    accumulation of phosphomycin, 168,
    169
HR 756, 44, 46
Hydrogen peroxide, 59
Hydroxyphenylazopyrimidines
    inhibitors of Gram-positive DNA
    polymerase III, 102, 103, 104
    reduction to active hydrazines, 102
    structures, 102
    unusual base-pairing with pyrimidine
    bases, 103
Hypochlorite, 3, 59

IdUrd, see 5-Iododeoxyuridine
Immunological control of infectious
    disease, 2
IMP
    conversion to adenylosuccinic acid, 81,
    83
    conversion to xanthylic acid, 81, 85
IMP-dehydrogenase from *Bacillus subtilis,*
    inhibition by mycophenolic acid, 85
IMP-NAD oxidoreductase, see IMP-
    dehydrogenase
Indolmycin, 117, 118
Infectious disease, effects of
    control, 1

Influenza A$_2$, prophylaxis with
    amantadine, 157
INH, see Isonicotinic hydrazide
Inhibition of peptidoglycan biosynthesis,
    evidence of this type of antibacterial
    action, 38
Inhibitors of protein synthesis
    effects on eukaryotic cells, 135, 136
    effects on nucleic acid synthesis, 134,
    135
    effects on polysomes, 133, 134
    effects on prokaryotic cells, 132, 133
Initiation of protein biosynthesis, 113
Intercalation of DNA by planar molecules,
    86 ff.
Inteferon, promise in treatment of viral
    infections, 157
Iodine, 3
5-Iododeoxyuridine
    interference with DNA synthesis and
    function, 106, 107
    structure, 106
    use in herpes infections, 106, 156
Ionization of antibacterial agents, effect
    on penetration into bacterial cells, 161
Ionophores binding divalent ions, 72
Ionophoric antibiotics
    effects on potassium transport, 70
    promotion of potassium flux in
    artificial membranes, 70
    relative affinities for sodium and
    potassium, 71
    structural requirements for activity,
    70, 71
Ipecacuanha root, 2
Iron-chelating antibiotics, 150
Iron-chelating growth factors, 151
Isoniazid, see Isonicotinic hydrazide
Isonicotinic hydrazide, 149, 150
    causes lowering of NAD in myco-
    bacteria, 150
    effect on mycolic acid biosynthesis, 150
    inhibition of C-24 acid Δ^5 desaturase,
    150
Isoprenyl phosphate (C$_{55}$), see
    Undecaprenyl phosphate
Isosteres, 140
Isotetracycline, 125

Kanamycin
    acetylation, 192, 193
    adenylation, 192, 193
    biochemical action, 121
    phosphorylation, 192, 193
    resistance to, 192, 193, 194
    structure, 122
Kasugamycin, site of ribosomal resistance,
    195
KDO, (2-keto-3-deoxymanno octulosonic
    acid), see 3-Deoxy-D-*manno*-
    octulosonic acid
β-Ketoacyl acyl carrier protein synthetase,
    inhibited by cerulenin, 55
Koch, Robert, 3

L-forms
  enhanced sensitivity of to anti-
    bacterial agents, 163
  resistance to antibiotics affecting
    peptidoglycan synthesis, 38
β-Lactamases, 45
  chemical approaches to the problem
    of, 187, 188
  Gram-negative, 186, 187
  Gram-positive, 186
  mechanism, 50, 185
  origin, 188, 189
  relationship to carboxypeptidases and
    transpeptidases, 50
  synthesis, 186
Leprosy, treatment with 4, 4'-diaminodi-
  phenylsulphone, 139
Lincomycin
  binding to ribosomes, 130
  clinical use, 130
  effect on yeast cells, 135
  inhibition of transpeptidation, 130
  structure, 130
Linear polymer formation in
  peptidoglycan biosynthesis, 30
Lipid A, component of lipopolysaccharide,
  26, 27
Lipopolysaccharide, in *S. typhimurium*
  wall, 27
Lipopolysaccharide of Gram-negative
  cells, importance in permeability
  of outer envelope to antibacterial
  agents, 163, 164, 165
Lipoprotein
  in *E. coli* wall, 27, 37
  occurrence in various Gram-negative
    bacteria, 38
  structure, 37
Lister, Joseph, 3
Lysogenic phages, induction of by
  mitomycin, 97

M & B 693, *see* Sulphapyridine
MBC, *see* Methyl benzimidazole
  carbamate
Macromolecular synthesis, interference
  by antimicrobial agents, 16
Macrotetrolides, 70
  structure of potassium complex, 71
Magnesium
  displaced from cytoplasmic membrane
    by polymyxin, 66
  release from mitochondria by A23187,
    72
  significance in Gram-negative
    bacterial wall, 26, 163
  tetracycline and, 126
Malaria
  treatment with folic acid antagonists,
    143
  treatment with mepacrine, 8, 9
  treatment with quinine, 2
Mapharsen
  metabolite of salvarsan, 8

structure, 6
Matrix protein of outer membrane, 26
Mecillinam, 44, 45
  mainly bound to protein 2 of
    cytoplasmic membrane, 53
Melarsen, inhibition of phosphokinase
  in trypanosomes, 154
Membrane, site of DNA replication, 86
Mepacrine, 8
Mercuric chloride
  as antiseptic, 3
  failure as systemic antibacterial, 4
Mercury salts and derivatives, 59
Messenger RNA, binding to ribosomes,
  113
Metabolism, in activation of antimicrobial
  compounds, 7, 8
Metabolite intermediates, accumulation
  during antibacterial action, 15
Methicillin, 44, 45
  substrate for β-lactamase, 187
Methisazone
  prophylactic use in smallpox, 157
  structure, 157
  suggested biochemical action, 157
Methotrexate, 143
Methyl benzimidazole carbamate,
  fungicide, 153
Methylbenzoquate
  inhibition of respiration in coccidial
    mitochondria, 155
  structure, 156
5-Methyl tryptophan, mechanism of
  resistance to, 200
24-Methylene dihydrolanosterol,
  demethylation blocked by diclo-
    butrazole, 152
L-N-Methylvaline, in actinomycin D, 90,
  92
Methylene blue, 5
Metronidazole, 155
  activity perhaps due to reduction
    product, 156
  structure, 156
Miconazole
  action against *Candida,* 152
  structure, 153
Microbial resistance, 172 ff.
  recognition by Ehrlich, 8
Minimal enzyme, of RNA polymerase,
  100, 101
Minocycline, penetration into bacteria,
  167
Minor groove of DNA, importance in
  DNA-actinomycin D interaction, 92
Misreading of genetic code, induction
  by aminoglycosides, 119, 120, 121
Mitochondria, 55S ribosomes, 110, 111
Mitomycin
  activation, 97
  biochemical effects on cells, 97
  clinical use, 95
  cross-linking of DNA, 95, 96, 97, 98
Mode of action of antimicrobial agents, 15

methods of study, 14
Moenocinol, structure, 42
Moenomycin, 42
Monensin
    as coccidiostat, 72
    preferential binding to sodium, 71
    sodium complex, 72
    structure, 71
    tonnage production, 72
    used to improve food conversion in
        ruminants, 72
Monoiodoamphenicol, interaction
    with ribosomal proteins, 127
mRNA, *see* Messenger RNA
Mucopeptide, *see* Peptidoglycan
Muramic acid, 29
Murein, *see* peptidoglycan
Mutations
    drug-resistance and, 173, 174, 175
    types of, 173, 174
Mycobacteria, lipids in cell wall, 24, 36
Mycobacterial infections, treatment by
    synthetic antibacterials, 10
Mycolic acid, linkage to peptidoglycan
    in mycobacteria, 37
Mycolic acid biosynthesis, inhibition by
    INH, 150
Mycophenolic acid
    antimitotic action, 85
    inhibition of purine nucleotide
        synthesis by, 85
    structure, 84
Mycoplasmas
    outside usual Gram stain classification,
        22
    resistance to antibiotics affecting
        peptidoglycan synthesis, 38
    sensitivity to polyene antibiotics
        depends on sterol content of
        membrane, 75, 76

NAD$^+$, oxidation of IMP by, 85
Nalidixic acid
    clinical use, 104
    inhibitor of DNA synthesis, 104,
        105
    resistance, 104
    structure, 104
Neomycin
    biochemical action, 121
    biochemical mechanisms of inactiva-
        tion, 192, 193, 194
    structure, 123
Nigericin
    exchange of potassium and hydrogen
        ions, 72
    preferential binding of potassium, 71
Nitrofuran antibacterials
    inhibition of initiation of mRNA
        formation, 150
    mutagenic properties, 150
    probable activation by reduction, 150
Nitrofurantoin, 149, 150
Nocardicin A, 44, 46

Nonactin, 68, 71
Norleucine, 117
Novobiocin
    clinical use, 105
    inhibition of DNA synthesis, 105
    structure, 105
Nucleases, appearance of, in mitomycin
    treated cells, 97
Nucleic acid
    disturbance of template function of,
        80, 85
    inhibitors of biosynthesis of, 79 ff.
Nucleic acid polymerases, as targets
    for drug action, 97 ff.
Nucleic acid synthesis, effects of
    inhibitors of protein synthesis on,
        134, 135
Nucleotide pentapeptide, 30
Nucleotides, inhibition of biosynthesis,
    80, 81, 82, 83, 84, 85
Nutrient receptors, in outer bacterial
    membrane, 28, 164, 165
Nystatin
    clinical use, 75
    interaction with sterols containing
        a conjugated diene, 76
    structure, 75

Octapeptins, 65
Oligomycin
    causes decreased proton permeability
        of membranes, 149
    inhibition of adenosine triphosphatase,
        148
    inhibition of coupled respiration, 147
    structure, 148
Oligomycin sensitivity-conferring
    protein, link between ATPase and
    mitochondrial membrane, 148
Oligopeptide permease, of bacterial cells,
    169
OSCP, *see* Oligomycin sensitivity-
    conferring protein
Outer envelope of Gram-negative cells,
    as a permeability barrier to anti-
    bacterial drugs, 162, 163, 164, 165
Outer membrane in Gram-negative
    rods, 24, 164, 165
    anchorage to peptidoglycan layer, 28
    asymetry, 26
    hydrophobic layer, 26
    phospholipid, 26
    selective permeability, 26
    structural proteins, 26
    transport proteins, 28
Oxidative phosphorylation
    association with membrane-bound
        ATPase, 148
    inhibition by oligomycin, 147
Oxolinic acid
    inhibitor of DNA synthesis, 104, 105
    resistance, 104
    structure, 105
Oxygen uptake, inhibition by antimycin, 145

Oxytetracycline, structure, 123
Ozone, 59

Parafuchsin, resistance in trypanosomes, 8
Park nucleotides, 28
Park, J.T., 28
Pasteur, Louis, 3, 4
Penicillin
  accumulation of nucleotides in
  S. aureus, 28
  antibacterial action, 47
  derivatives stable to penicillinases,
  45, 187
  discovery, 10
  effect on cell ultrastructure, 48
  effect on *E. coli,* 52
  inhibition of peptidoglycan cross-
  linking, 47
  isolation and purification, 11
  modern treatment for syphilis, 5
  precursors in fermentation medium, 43
  rigid structure, 52
  structural resemblance to D-alanyl-
  D-alanine end group, 51
Penicillin G, 43
  inactivation by acid, 43
Penicillin binding proteins
  in *E. coli* cytoplasmic membrane, 52,
  53
  differing functions, 53
Penicillin V, stability to acid, 43
Penicillinase, 45, 185 (*see also* β-lactamase)
Penicillins
  activity of 6-methoxy derivatives, 52
  antibacterial spectrum and medical
  uses, 43, 45
  effects on Gram-negative bacteria, 45,
  52
  6-methyl, lacking antibacterial
  activity, 52
  semi-synthetic, active against Gram-
  negative bacteria, 45
  semi-synthetic, resistant to β-lactamase,
  45, 187
  structure, 44
  tight binding to serine at active centre
  of carboxypeptidase, 51
Penicillium, source of penicillin, 10
Penta-*N*-benzyl polymyxin, preferential
  activity against Gram-positive
  bacteria, 65
Pentaglycine group, in peptidoglycan
  biosynthesis, 31
Peptide bond formation, 114
  inhibition by chloramphenicol, 128
Peptide chain termination and release, 115
Peptide permease, of bacterial cells, 169
Peptidoglycan
  biosynthesis of linear polysaccharide,
  30
  biosynthesis of pentapeptide side
  chain, 29
  catabolism during cell growth, 35
  cross-linking pattern, 33

  differences between bacterial strains,
  35
  extending group, 31
  function, 23, 24
  hydrolysis products, 28
  isolation, 28
  linkage with lipoprotein in *E. coli*
  wall, 37
  linkage with teichoic acid in *S. aureus,*
  36
  structure and biosynthesis, 28
  thickness in Gram-positive bacterial
  wall, 22
  thinness and flexibility in Gram-
  negative bacterial wall, 24
  type B, having linkage through
  D-glutamic group, 35
Peptidoglycan biosynthesis
  amidation of carboxyl group of
  D-glutamic acid, 31
  cross-linking, 33
  function of the 'acceptor', 31
  in Gram-negative rods, differences
  between wall extension and septum
  formation, 36
  inhibition by antibiotics, 38
  transpeptidation in cross-linking
  process, 33
  unlinked linear polymer in bacteria
  treated with penicillin, 49
Peptidyl transferase
  inhibition by chloramphenicol, 128
  in peptide bond formation, 114
Periplasmic space, 24
Permeability of cytoplasmic membrane
  caused by antiseptics, 60
Permeability of microbial cells to drugs,
  159 ff.
  enhancement by ethylenediaminetetraacetic acid, 163
  enhancement by polyenes, 170
  loss of as mechanism of drug
  resistance, 196, 197, 198
Phage receptor sites, associated with
  transport proteins, 28
Phage transduction of drug resistance,
  174, 176, 177
Pharmacological biochemistry of
  antimicrobial agents, 13
Phenanthridines
  binding to DNA, 89
  inhibition of nucleic acid synthesis
  by, 95
  medical use, 89
  structure (ethidium), 88
  vital staining, 89
Phenazine-*N*-oxides, 149
Phenol, as antiseptic in surgery, 3
Phenols, 4
  as antiseptics, 60
  inactivity in systemic infections, 9
Phenoxyacetic acid, as penicillin
  precursor, 43
Phenoxymethyl penicillin, 43, **44**

Phenylacetic acid, as penicillin precursor, 43
Phenylacetylglycine, enzymic degradation product of benzyl penicillin, 50
Phosphatidylethanolamine, in outer membrane, 26
Phosphatidylglycerol in outer membrane, 26
Phosphokinase in trypanosomes, inhibition by melarsen, 154
Phospholipid synthesis, inhibited by cerulenin, 55
Phospholipids, in Gram-negative walls, 26
Phosphomycin, 39
    uptake by bacterial cells, 168, 169
Phosphonomycin, *see* Phosphomycin
Phosphorylation of aminoglycosides, 192, 193, 194
Physical properties of antimicrobial agents, importance in determining penetration into cells, 160, 161
Piericidin, blocks link between NAD dehydrogenases and respiratory pathway, 147
Plasmids, 88
    in drug resistance, 176 ff.
Polyamine permease, role in amino-glycoside uptake by bacteria, 168
Polyene antibiotics
    action on fungal infections, 75
    basis of selectivity, 75
    effects on red cells, 76
    increase the permeability of fungal membranes, 76
    interaction with sterols to form a membrane pore, 76
    molecular conformation, 76
    toxicity, 75, 76
    structure and use, 75
    synergism with other antifungal agents, 170
Polymyxin
    binding to bacteria, 65
    'blistering' effect on outer membrane, 66
    effect of on permeability of cytoplasmic membrane, 66
    fluorescent adduct used to show membrane binding, 65
    increases permeability of *Pseudomonas aeruginosa,* 65
    low concentrations inhibit bacterial respiration, 65
    nature of binding to cytoplasmic membrane, 66
    pentabenzyl derivative, showing reversed bacterial selectivity, 65
    use and antibacterial action, 65
Polymyxin B_1, structure, 64
Polyoxin D, structure, 55
Polyoxins, inhibition of chitin biosynthesis, 56
Polypeptide antibiotics, 64

importance of cyclic structure, 67
Polysomes, 133
    effect of inhibitors of protein synthesis on, 134
Population explosion, contribution of antimicrobial agents, 1
Pores
    of outer bacterial membrane, 161, 164
    permeability function, 161, 164
Porfiromycin
    biochemical action, 95, 96, 97
    structure, 96
Porins, 26
Potassium, complexes with macro-tetrolides, 71
Potassium ions
    bacterial uptake inhibited by chlorhexidine at low concentration, 62
    leakage caused by antiseptics, 60
    permeability of cell membranes in presence of ionophoric antibiotics, 67, 71
    preferential binding to ionophoric antibiotics, 70
    promotion of flux through artificial membranes by ionophoric antibiotics, 70
Proflavine, 88
Proguanil
    metabolic conversion to a dihydrotriazine, 143
    structure, 143
Prontosil rubrum, 9, 138
Protein F1, solubilized ATPase from mitochondria, 148
Protein binding, and activity of anti-microbial agents, 13
Protein biosynthesis
    inhibition, 110 ff.
    interrelationship with nucleic acid synthesis, 134, 135
    stages in, 111, 112, 113, 114, 115
Protein conferring sensitivity to streptomycin, 120
Proteins
    in Gram-negative outer membrane, 26
    in Gram-positive walls, 24
Proteins conferring sensitivity to chloramphenicol, 127
Proteins conferring sensitivity to erythromycin, 128, 129
Protoplasts, absorption of antiseptics, 59
Protozoal diseases, chemotherapy, 89, 154
Psicofuranine
    clinical use, 83
    inhibition of purine nucleotide synthesis by, 83
    mechanism of resistance to, 200
    structure, 84
Purine nucleotides
    biosynthetic sequence, 81
    inhibition of synthesis, 80 ff.
Puromycin
    importance of, 115

structural analogues, 116, 117
structural resemblance to aminoacyl
tRNA, 115, 116
structure, 115
termination of protein biosynthesis,
115, 116
Puromycin reaction
effect of inhibitors of protein
biosynthesis, 117
inhibition by chloramphenicol, 128
inhibition by erythromycin, 129
inhibition by lincomycin, 130
Pyrimethamine, 143
affinity for dihydrofolate reductase
from *Plasmodium vinckei,* 144
Pyrophosphatase releasing membrane
lipid phosphate, inhibition by
bacitracin, 54

Quinacrine, *see* Mepacrine
Quinine, 2
Quinoxaline antibiotics, 92, 93
Quinoxaline *N*-oxides, possible
interference with DNA synthesis, 149

R-factors
classification, 178
discovery, 177
nature, 179, 180
number of copies, 181
relationship to F-factors, 181
role in transfer of drug-resistance,
177, 181, 182, 183, 184
Radioactive labelling in study of antimicrobial agents, 13
Receptors, in resistant micro-organisms, 8
Receptors for drugs, Ehrlich's theory, 6
Recombination, in R-factors, 179
Release factors, role in peptide chain
termination, 115
Replica plating technique, 173, 174, 175
Resistance, 18, 172 ff.
approaches to the control of, 201,
202, 203
biochemical mechanisms, 184 ff.
genetic basis, 172, 173, 174
Respiratory pathway, inhibition by
antibiotics, 145, 146
Ribitol teichoic acid, structure, 23, 37
Ribosomal cycle, diagram, 112
Ribosomal proteins, 111
Ribosomal RNA, 111
Ribosome
subunits, 110, 111
types, 110, 111
Rifampicin
inhibition of RNA polymerase, 100,
101
resistance to, 100, 195
structure, 99
Rifamycins, 97
resistance to, 100, 195
Ringworm, treated with griseofulvin, 152
Ristocetin, 42

RNA, effect of inhibitors of protein
biosynthesis on, 135
RNA biosynthesis
effects of inhibition on protein
biosynthesis, 16, 119
effects of mitomycin, 97
inhibition by actinomycin D, 95
inhibition by intercalating dyes, 95
inhibition by rifamycins, 97, 98, 100,
101
inhibition by streptolydigin, 101, 102
inhibition by streptovaricins, 97, 98,
100, 101
RNA chains, inhibition of initiation and
elongation, 100, 101
RNA polymerase
binding to DNA, 100
inhibition by antimicrobial drugs, 100,
101
streptolydigin and, 101
streptovaricins and, 99, 100, 101
subunit structure, 100
rifampicin and, 99, 100, 101
Rutamycin, 147

Sacculus, 35
Salvage pathways, role in drug-resistance,
199
Salvarsan, 5, 6
effect on motility of spirochetes, 7
metabolism to mapharsen, 8
Screening, in the search for anti-
microbial drugs, 7
Sedimentation coefficient of DNA,
effect of intercalating dyes, 86, 87
Selectivity in antimicrobial action, 17
'Septrin', *see* Cotrimoxazole
Septum formation, effect of penicillins, 48
Sex pili, role in bacterial conjugation,
181, 182, 183
Sideramines, 151
Sideromycins, 150
antagonism of transport by
sideramines, 151
nature of bacterial toxicity, 151
uptake by bacterial cells, 167
Sigma factor, RNA polymerase and, 100
Sleeping sickness, first cured by atoxyl, 5
Smallpox, prophylaxis with methisazone,
157
Spectinomycin
biochemical action, 122
structure, 122
Spheroplasts, 38
absorption of antiseptics, 59
Spirochetes, action of salvarsan, 7
Stabilization of Gram-negative outer
membrane by Mg^{2+} and Ca^{2+}, 26
Sterilants, 58
Sterol biosynthesis blocked by fungicides,
152
Sterols
absence in most bacterial membranes,
75

in fungal membrane, binding of polyene antibiotics, 75
Streptolydigin, inhibitor of bacterial RNA polymerase, 101, 102
Streptomycin
    adenylation of, 193
    antibacterial action, 118, 133
    bacterial dependence on, 133
    binding to ribosomes, 120
    clinical use, 118
    conflicting views on mode of action, 14
    discovery, 118
    disruption of bacterial cytoplasmic membrane, 133
    effect on *Chlamydomonas,* 135
    effect on *Euglena,* 135
    effects on protein biosynthesis, 119, 120, 121
    hazards of use, 118
    induction of codon misreading, 119
    mechanism of bactericidal action, 133
    mode of entry into bacterial cells, 168
    phosphorylation, 193
    resistance to, 193
    ribosomal stability and, 133
    site of ribosomal action, 120, 121
    structure, 118
Streptovaricins, inhibitors of bacterial RNA polymerase, 99, 100, 101
Strominger, Jack Leonard, 28, 47, 51
Sulphadiazine, 138
    structure, 139
Sulphadimidine, 138
    structure, 139
Sulphafurazole, 138
    structure, 139
Sulphamethoxazole, 144
    structure, 139
Sulphanilamide, 9
    metabolic product from Prontosil rubrum, 138
Sulphanilic acid, inhibition of *in vitro* synthesis of dihydropteroic acid, 140
Sulphapyridine, 138, 139
Sulphonamide analogues of dihydropteroate, lack of antibacterial significance, 141
Sulphonamide antibacterials, 138
    as substrates competing with *p*-aminobenzoate, 141
    competitive antagonism of action by *p*-aminobenzoic acid, 140
    effects on intermediary metabolism, 145
    favourable factors in their practical success, 142
    inhibition of *in-vitro* synthesis of dihydropteroic acid, 140
    isosteres of *p*-aminobenzoic acid, 140
    mechanisms of resistance to, 198, 201
    medical uses, 138, 144
    structural requirements for activity, 138
Supersensitive bacterial mutants, 164
Suramin, 8, 9

specificity of structure, 154
Synthetic antibacterials, use in various infections, 10
Syphilis, treatment by salvarsan, 5

Target site, interaction with the antimicrobial agent, 17
Teichoic acid, 23, 36
    labile linkage to peptidoglycan, 36
    possible function, 24
    possible influence on drug penetration, 163
    structure, 37
Teichoic acid biosynthesis, link with peptidoglycan synthesis, 36
Teichuronic acid, 23
Termination, in protein biosynthesis, 115
Terminator codons, 115
Tetracyclines, 123
    active uptake by bacterial cells, 123, 166, 167
    antibacterial action, 123
    binding to ribosomes, 124
    chelating activity, 126
    effects on eukaryotic protein synthesis, 123
    inhibition of aminoacyl tRNA-ribosome interaction, 123, 124
    mechanism of resistance to, 197, 198
    ribosomal site of action, 124
    selectivity of action, 123
    structure-activity relationships, 125, 126
    structures, 123, 125
Tetrahydrofolate biosynthesis, double blockage, 145
Thiamine, uptake inhibited by amprolium, 155
Thienamycin, 44, 46
Thiol groups, possible involvement in antimicrobial action of arsenicals, 14
Thymineless death, induced by sulphonamides or trimethoprim, 145
Tipper, D.J., 28, 47
Tobramycin, resistance, 194
Tolyl-1-naphthylamine-8-sulphonic acid, *see* Tolyl-peri acid
Tolylperi acid
    in demonstration of permeability of bacteria, 61, 65
    shows bacterial permeability induced by polymyxin, 65
Toxophore, 7
Transduction, spread of drug-resistance by, 174, 176, 177
Transfer factor, *see* R-factors
Transfer RNA
    binding to ribosomes, 113
    translocation in protein biosynthesis, 114
Transformation, spread of drug-resistance by, 174
Transition point of membranes, effect on transport of ions by valinomycin and gramicidin A, 74

Translocation
 inhibition by cycloheximide, 132
 inhibition by erythromycin, 129, 130
 inhibition by fusidic acid, 131
 in protein biosynthesis, 114
Transpeptidase
 difficulty of solubilization and
  isolation, 35, 49
 inhibition by penicillin, 47
 in peptidoglycan cross-linking, 33
Transpeptidase action, compared with
  carboxypeptidase action, 49
Transpeptidase activity in soluble
  carboxypeptidases, 49
Transpeptidases in peptidoglycan
  biosynthesis, membrane suspension, 47
Transposons, 178, 179
Tréfouël, J., 9
Triforin
 sterol biosynthesis blocked at C-14
  demethylation step, 152
 structure, 153
Trimethoprim
 resistance, 199
 selective inhibition of dihydrofolate
  reductase from bacteria, 144
 structure, 143
Triostin A
 interaction with DNA, 92, 93
 structure, 93
tRNA, *see* Transfer RNA
Trypan red, 5
 resistance in trypanosomes, 8
Trypanosomes
 dependence on phosphokinase, 154
 kinetoplast DNA and intercalating
  molecules, 88, 154
 surface charge, 155
Trypanosomiasis
 cured by trypan red, 5
 treated with arsenious oxide, 4
 treatment with ethidium, 89
 treatment with suramin, 8
Tuberculosis
 treatment with *p*-aminosalicylic acid,
  139
 treatment with INH, 150
 treatment with synthetic compounds,
  10
Tunicamycin
 inhibition of carbohydrate
  polymerization, 43
 structure, 42
Typhoid fever, treatment by chloramphenicol, 126
Tyrocidin A
 molecular topography, 67

 structure, 64
Tyrocidins, 66
 cause fall in membrane potential of
  N.crassa, 64
 effects on bacterial permeability, 64

Ubiquinol-cytochrome *c* oxido-reductase,
  inhibition by antimycin, 147
UDP-*N*-acetyl muramyl pentapeptide, in
  bacteria treated with drugs affecting
  peptidoglycan synthesis, 39
Uncoupling agents, prevention of action
  of oligomycin, 147
Undecaprenyl phosphate in peptidoglycan
  biosynthesis, 31
Undecaprenyl pyrophosphatase, 33
 inhibition by bacitracin, 54
Uptake of antimicrobial drugs, 159 ff.
 exploitation in design of new drugs,
  169, 170, 171
Uridine nucleotides of *N*-acetyl muramic
  acid, accumulation during action of
  inhibitors of peptidoglycan biosynthesis
  biosynthesis, 38
UDP-*N*-acetylmuramic acid biosynthesis,
  29

Valinomycin, 68
 mechanism of complex formation, 70
 a mobile carrier of ions, 70
 optical configuration of constituent
  amino acids, 69
 structure, 68, 69
 turnover number, 70
Vancomycin
 binding to D-alanyl-D-alanyl group, 42
 binding to bacterial walls, 42
 structure, 42
 uses and toxicity, 42
Viable count, 59
Virus chemotherapy, 106, 107, 156
Viscosity of DNA solutions
 effect of actinomycin D, 90
 effect of intercalating compounds, 86,
  87
Vital stains, 5, 89

Waksman, Selman, A., 11

X-ray analysis of deoxyguanosine-
  actinomycin D complex, 91, 92
Xanthosine, 84
XMP, amination, 81, 83
XMP aminase
 desensitization, 83
 inhibition, 83
XMP, inhibition of biosynthesis, 85